MW01096419

The Mumbo Jumbo Fix hits a home run! [An E]xcellent book by an eminently qualified author who has lived it. Easy to read, organized with many valuable insights and vignettes.... Patients who read this book will end up improving their chances of the best outcome the profession offers.
—Dominick Addario, MD, Psychiatrist, Diplomate, American Board of Psychiatry and Neurology, Distinguished Life Fellow, American Psychiatric Association, Health Sciences Clinical Professor, University of California San Diego

Easy to read, and systematic approach to maximizing on first principles of communication in healthcare, and more broadly.... The book does not take itself too seriously, with a smattering of cartoons thrown in to make the subject light-hearted, but relevant and relatable. I highly recommend this book to all physicians, nurses, and others who support them.
—Javed Siddiqi, HBSc, MD, DPhil (Oxon), FRCSC, FACS, FAANS, Neurosurgeon, Chief of Neurosurgery, ARMC, RUHS, RCH & DRMC, Professor & Chair, Dept of Surgery, California University of Science & Medicine, Founding Journal Editor, *Contemporary Reviews in Neurology & Neurosurgery*, President Elect, California Association of Neurological Surgeons

The Mumbo Jumbo Fix is a long overdue resource for healthcare professionals, patients, and families. This book presents communication strategies in a clear and often humorous format.... Medical and nursing programs should include this book as a required text for improved communications skills.
—Elsa L. Murdoch, DNP, MSN, RN, CPHRM, Assistant Professor, RN-BSN Program Director, Azusa Pacific University

Who better to see the many problems of doctor-patient-nurse communication than an experienced medical malpractice attorney? Mike Grace has seen and heard it all. *The Mumbo Jumbo Fix* is loaded with entertaining and revealing stories of miscommunication between doctors and nurses and between both and patients.... It is a must read for both health professionals in training and those with experience.
—Joseph E. Scherger, MD, MPH, Family Practice Physician, Primary Care 365 Physician Core Faculty, Family Medicine Residency Program, Eisenhower Medical Center, Clinical Professor of Family Medicine, Keck School of Medicine, University of Southern California

An absolute must read for anyone who wants to improve communication and patient relationships. A comprehensive communication guide. Even the most seasoned healthcare professional will benefit from reading this book.
—Nicholas Wade, BSN, MPH, CEAS, Public Health Nurse, West Bay Area Director of Employee Health Service & Workers Compensation, Sutter Health

....The book was very worthwhile, easy to read, concise, and entertaining which holds all healthcare workers' attention. I appreciated the cartoons... I found myself smiling or laughing aloud at times. This book's subject has a role in the education of medical students and all healthcare workers.
—Lori J. Beck, DNP, Nurse Practitioner, Indiana University Health

....[V]ery eloquently written.... [W]itty comical illustrations.... [A]n easy read that can be read in one sitting or multiple sittings because you can pick right back up where you left off....
—Karen Seessengood, MSN, RN, CNOR, CST/CSFA, Nurse Perioperative Educator, Founder, Seessengood Perioperative Education and Consulting, Princeton, IN, Staff RN/Perioperative Educator, Surgery Department, Logansport Memorial Hospital

The Mumbo Jumbo Fix

The Mumbo Jumbo Fix

A Survival Guide for Effective Doctor-Patient-Nurse
Communication

Written and Illustrated by

Michael J. Grace, JD, CPHRM

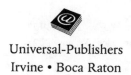

Universal-Publishers
Irvine • Boca Raton

The Mumbo Jumbo Fix:
A Survival Guide for Effective Doctor-Patient-Nurse Communication

For permission to photocopy or use material electronically from this work, please access www.copyright.com or contact the Copyright Clearance Center, Inc. (CCC) at 978-750-8400. CCC is a not-for-profit organization that provides licenses and registration for a variety of users. For organizations that have been granted a photocopy license by the CCC, a separate system of payments has been arranged.

Universal Publishers, Inc.
Irvine, California & Boca Raton, Florida • USA
www.Universal-Publishers.com
2021

ISBN: 978-1-62734-366-4 (pbk.)
ISBN: 978-1-62734-367-1 (ebk.)

Typeset by Medlar Publishing Solutions Pvt Ltd, India
Cover design by Jeremy Blanger

Library of Congress Cataloging-in-Publication Data

Names: Grace, Michael J., 1950-author.
Title: The mumbo jumbo fix : a survival guide for effective
    doctor-patient-nurse communication / written and illustrated by Michael J.
    Grace, JD, CPHRM.
Description: Irvine : Universal Publishers, [2021] | Includes
    bibliographical references.
Identifiers: LCCN 2021039076 (print) | LCCN 2021039077 (ebook) | ISBN
    9781627343664 (paperback) | ISBN 9781627343671 (ebook)
Subjects: LCSH: Communication in medicine. | Miscommunication. | Medical
    personnel and patient.
Classification: LCC R118 .G72 2021 (print) | LCC R118 (ebook) | DDC
    610.69/6--dc23
LC record available at https://lccn.loc.gov/2021039076
LC ebook record available at https://lccn.loc.gov/2021039077

About the Author

Michael J. Grace, JD, CPHRM

Mike is a licensed attorney and is designated by the American Hospital Association as a certified professional in healthcare risk management. He was a founding partner of Grace Hollis LLC, a San Diego based law firm, where he specialized in the defense of healthcare providers. After twenty years as the firm's lead trial attorney, he "retired" to pursue a new chapter in life as the Risk Manager and Patient Safety Officer at Desert Regional Medical Center, a large Southern California hospital. Currently he teaches communication and law to nurses in the University of California, Riverside's extension program.

His interest in communication and medicine was established at an early age. Mike was a high school debater and forensic champion. He went to San Diego State University on a debate scholarship where he majored in speech communication. He graduated with High Honors and went on to graduate school at the University of California, Davis to pursue a master's degree in the Department of Rhetoric. This was followed by a year on a Rotary Fellowship at the University of Stockholm's International Graduate School to study mass communication.

Mike returned to California for law school at the University of San Diego where he achieved a juris doctorate degree, followed by admission to the California and Nevada Bars. He quickly recognized he wanted to spend his legal career in the exciting intersection of law and medicine. Mike currently holds an "AV" rating from Martindale-Hubbell, the highest possible peer reviewed national attorney rating.

In private practice when not representing doctors, nurses and hospitals in the courtroom, Mike was teaching them. As an expert on healthcare communication, Mike has been a frequent invited lecturer to scores of healthcare groups throughout the State of California. He is passionate about his chosen field and enjoys enthusiastically sharing his experience. As entertainer Steven Colbert recognizes: "You can't really be passionately moderate. It's like wearing an 'extra medium'—it doesn't exist."

After years in the courtroom defending healthcare providers, Mike jumped at the chance to work inside a hospital system to improve communication and prevent medical errors. In his role of hospital administrative officer, Mike had primary responsibility for investigating every incident of injury and "near miss" to determine the root cause as well as institute and evaluate corrective actions plans to prevent future harm. This hospital experience reinforced the lessons learned from decades of defense legal work—miscommunication among doctors, nurses and patients was at the center of many problems within healthcare.

Mike lives in Palm Springs. When he's not traveling, Mike enjoys reading, photography and painting. His paintings have appeared in several art exhibitions in Southern California.

Mike would like to hear from you about your healthcare communication experiences. He can be reached at mikegraceart@gmail.com.

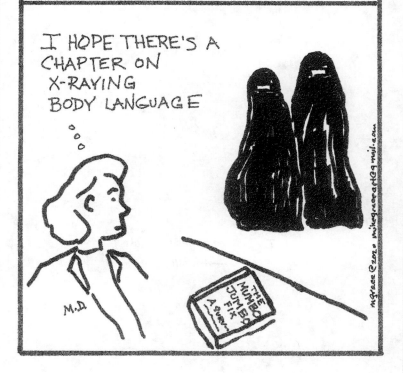

The gods too are fond of a joke.
—*Aristotle*

Table of Contents

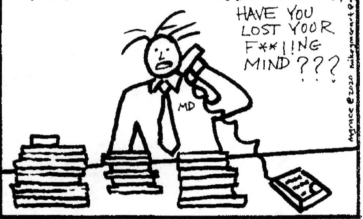

1
Where We Are

IN THIS CHAPTER

Patients learn miscommunication among healthcare participants—doctors, patients, and nurses—is the cause of most medical errors but they have usually been excluded as a target audience from books on the subject.

Nurses familiar with hospital education initiatives will recognize a continuing need for improved communication among all healthcare participants.

Doctors' ability to communicate effectively remains elusive despite the best of intentions, formal training, and clinical experience.

"He doesn't listen." "She didn't tell me." "I thought I understood."
"How many times do I have to say it?"
"Half the time I don't know what he's talking about."
"Why doesn't she just get to the point?"

As a hospital Risk Manager and Patient Safety Officer, every day I encountered the effects of linguistic mumbo jumbo within the healthcare system—meaningless, confusing, and ineffective communication among doctors, patients, and nurses. As a trial attorney defending healthcare providers, I regularly saw firsthand the legal consequences and harm of poor communication among healthcare participants. And as a speech communication major in undergraduate and graduate school and as a healthcare educator, I discovered there are evidence-based best practices which add value and clarity to any professional interpersonal exchange.

How did we get here? We talk at, over, and past one another when there are easily adopted and effective strategies for these essential interactions.

The Joint Commission, the accrediting organization for most American hospitals and healthcare organizations, has long focused on the link between effective communication and patient safety. Its sentinel event data identified communication as a root cause for almost two-thirds of the reported serious harm events between 2004 and 2016.[1] Ineffective communication continues to be among the top three root causes for serious adverse events along with leadership and human factors.[2]

It's not that medical and nursing schools ignore communication. On the contrary, all clinical programs teach the centrality of the effective exchange of information. Both for optimal patient outcomes and provider job satisfaction. Yet despite mandatory coursework and the best of intentions, healthcare providers graduate with improved but only average communication competence. Apparently, communication skills are getting lost in the press of mastering the growing mountain of required clinical skills. Nor does clinical experience improve communication; bad habits become ingrained and excellent interpersonal skills remain elusive.[3]

Hospitals and other large healthcare delivery systems know communication is vitally important. An alphabet soup of "easily remembered" mnemonic tools are regularly rolled out in an effort to boost patient satisfaction scores. But posters plastered on institutional walls touting "patient centered" communication become wallpaper. Consciously or subconsciously harried healthcare workers muddle on as they've always done trying to gather and relate critical healthcare information as rapidly as possible in a time pressurized environment.

Nor has self interest improved effective doctor-patient-nurse communication. Medical malpractice claims data show the failure of a physician to communicate with the patient or other providers is one of the most common and costly reasons for the initiation of litigation. A major study released in 2016 representing one-third of the total insurance market estimated communication

[1] The Joint Commission, "JC sentinel event data, root causes by event type 2004–2013," 2014 Oct 1, https://www.jointcommission.org/assets

[2] Cooke, M., "TeamSTEPPS for health care risk managers: Improving teamwork and communication," ASHRM Journal of Healthcare Risk Management, 2016; 36(3): 35,36

[3] Gilligan, C., Brubacher, S., Powell, M., "Assessing the training needs of medical students in patient information gathering," BMC Medical Education, 2020; 20:61

failures in U.S. hospitals and medical practices were responsible for 1,774 deaths and $1.7 billion in malpractice costs over the prior five years.[4]

Often the patient who sues is merely looking for understanding of an unexpected outcome. Unfortunately, many doctors shy away from addressing such problems out of ignorance, inertia or fear even when there may be a straight forward and medically sound explanation. So, patients pursue answers through the court system. Or as frequently happens, the physician did relate the proposed treatment's risks and benefits in an appropriate and timely fashion, but the message was not fully understood in the moment. And often the physician fails adequately to document the conversation. Again, the result is a lawsuit.

There is already much written on this vital subject of healthcare communication, usually in the form of academic studies and scholarly treatises. Hardly an approachable format for time-strapped professionals and busy lay people already overwhelmed with other concerns. *The Mumbo Jumbo Fix: A Survival Guide for Effective Doctor-Patient-Nurse Communication* is based on the author's extensive real-world experience as a medical malpractice trial lawyer, hospital administrative officer, and healthcare educator. It is intended as an accessible treatment of easily digestible bites of important information—practical strategies which can be read in any order as suits the reader's appetite.

Most books in the field take a siloed approach to fixing miscommunication within the healthcare industry. They typically focus on either doctors or nurses and largely ignore patient education. Yet all three groups—doctors, nurses, *and* patients—are its essential participants. Emphasizing only one group to the exclusion of the others is similar to family counseling where the therapist never brings the individual family members together as a group. Is it any surprise that miscommunication remains a major cause of medical errors? *The Mumbo Jumbo Fix* is literally the first healthcare communication book to get everyone on the same page!

---

[4] CRICO Strategies, "Malpractice risk in communication failures," 2015 Annual Benchmarking Report, Boston, MA: The Risk Management Foundation of the Harvard Medical Institutions, Inc., 2015

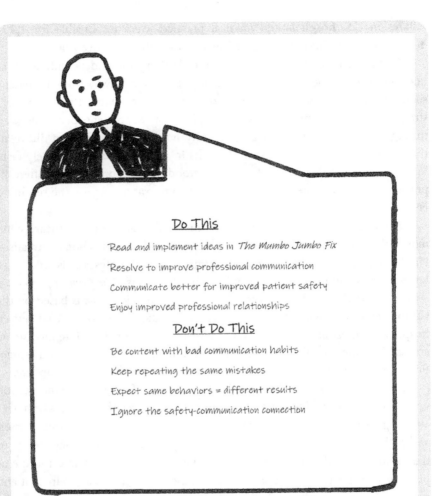

Do This

Read and implement ideas in *The Mumbo Jumbo Fix*

Resolve to improve professional communication

Communicate better for improved patient safety

Enjoy improved professional relationships

Don't Do This

Be content with bad communication habits

Keep repeating the same mistakes

Expect same behaviors = different results

Ignore the safety-communication connection

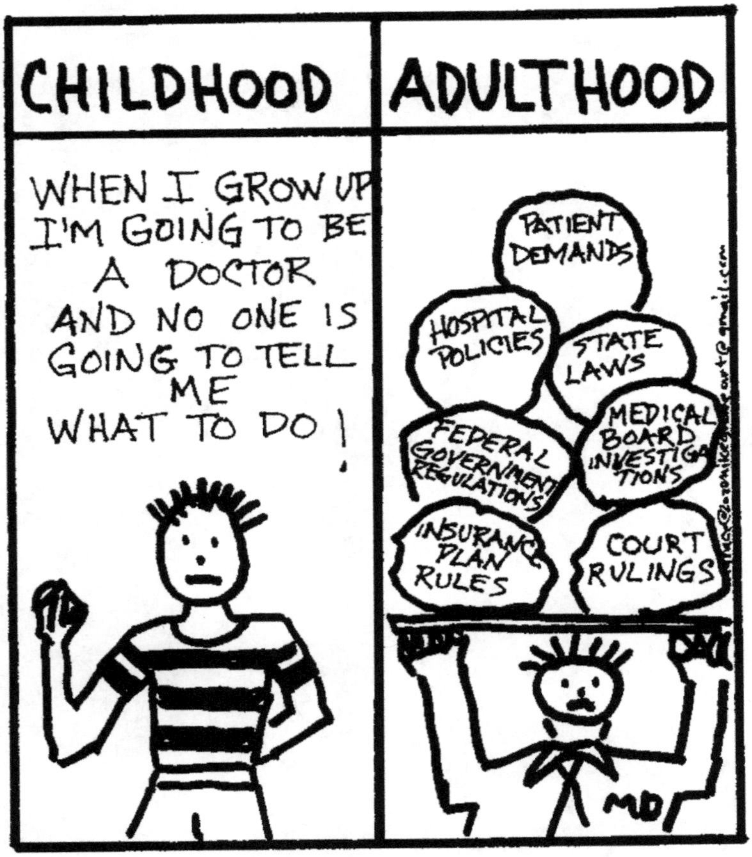
CHILDHOOD
ADULTHOOD
WHEN I GROW UP I'M GOING TO BE A DOCTOR AND NO ONE IS GOING TO TELL ME WHAT TO DO!
PATIENT DEMANDS
HOSPITAL POLICIES
STATE LAWS
FEDERAL GOVERNMENT REGULATIONS
MEDICAL BOARD INVESTIGATIONS
INSURANCE PLAN RULES
COURT RULINGS
MD

2
We Once Knew It All

IN THIS CHAPTER

Patients discover the key to effective communication is a skill taught when they were young, the same early education received by healthcare professionals.

Nurses and other healthcare providers learn they can reshape their professional lives through enhanced communication skills.

Doctors recognize they can improve patient outcomes by adopting evidence-based best communication practices.

The essence of excellent and effective communication is not mysterious, and it's easily attainable. You already know it. You learned it in the first grade.[5]

- Show respect
- Listen carefully
- Speak clearly
- Make eye contact
- Talk one at a time
- Avoid shouting
- Tell the truth
- Try to see the other side

---

[5] Morin, A., "Important Social Skills for First Grade," Very Well Family, 2020 Sept 17, https://www.verywellfamily.com/social-skills-that-are-important-for-1st-grade-620955

But what happened? We grew up. We became important. We got busy. We grew impatient. We got tired—of the demands, the expectations, the rules, the disrespect, and the stupidity. And we became fearful—and perhaps resentful—of change, the unknown and the loss of control. But as the rapper Tupac Shakur reminds us, "Things change. That's the way it is."

The good news is through effective communication we have the power to reshape our personal and professional lives. While there is some truth in the maxim "one cannot control anyone else," there is also truth in the knowledge "one can choose to control oneself and how to respond to others." And, frankly, there are even some evidence-based ways predictably and positively to affect others' communication behaviors. Enhanced doctor-patient-nurse relationships will lead to improved patient outcomes, greater job satisfaction, less work-related stress, and better time management.[6]

As Aristotle, the Greek philosopher and rhetorician, observed 2400 years ago: "A good relationship starts with good communication."

---

[6] Haq, C., Steele, D., Marchand, L., Seibert, C., Brody, D., "Integrating the Art and Science of Medical Practice: Innovations in Teaching Medical Communications Skills," Family Medicine, 2004 Jan; 36 Suppl: S43

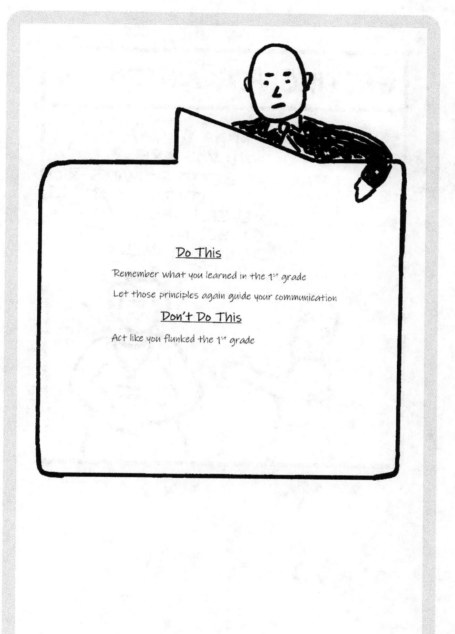

Do This

Remember what you learned in the 1ˢᵗ grade

Let those principles again guide your communication

Don't Do This

Act like you flunked the 1ˢᵗ grade

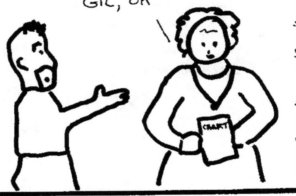

3
The Importance of a Name

IN THIS CHAPTER

Patients recognize the dignity of respectfully being called by name.

Nurses are reminded to address patients by their formal name until given permission to use a first name.

Doctors create a positive impression by calling patients by name, looking them in the eye while smiling, and remembering the name on subsequent encounters.

We all know it is hard to recover from a bad first impression. Knowing your patient's name is an important first positive step. Always verify the name in the chart before walking into the room. And every time thereafter. Make sure the patient you expect to see is in fact the one perched on your exam table!

Knowing the name is not enough. Use the name as you greet the patient. "A pleasure to meet you, Mrs. Padilla." And smile sincerely, looking the patient in the eye, as you say her name. Everyone wants to be acknowledged and recognized; no one wants to feel invisible. As motivational speaker Dale Carnegie famously said: "A person's name is to him or her the sweetest and most important sound in any language."

If you aren't sure how to pronounce the name, don't be shy about asking for clarification. Repeat the name as stated and make a mental phonetic note (and a written one later.) PA DI YA. Awkward second encounters are avoidable.

Knowing the patient's name on a subsequent visit tells the patient you thought she was special and took the time to remember her name.[7]

Until you have been given permission to use the patient's first name, keep it formal. While we live in a casual society and it's likely the patient will correct you by immediately sharing her first name, the display of initial respect will not go unnoticed. If the patient wants to be informal, take your cue. "Ok, Maria, thank you."

These rules of formality are especially important for young doctors interacting with older patients. Keeping it courteous and professional will always score brownie points, even with the most easy-going patients.

Now it's your turn to share your name. And any funny pronunciations. "Hello, I'm Dr. Derek Rajaputra. But most of my patients find it easier just to call me Dr. Raj." Just because the patient wants you to call her by a first name doesn't mean you have to do the same. Unless, the rare egalitarian patient is insistent, and then what's been good for Goose Maria should be good for Gander Derek.

Formal titles are less problematic within nursing where most nurses informally use first names, typically printed on a badge. It's natural for patients to use the badge first name. But like physicians, nurses should always begin addressing a patient with the appropriate respectful title and surname unless directed otherwise.

---

[7] Davis, L., "The Power of Using Someone's Name," The Native Idealist, 2017 Aug 10, https://www.goodmenproject.com/featured-content/the-power-of-using-someones-name-Idvs/

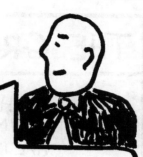

Do This

Know the patient's name

Use the patient's name

Greet the patient with a sincere smile

Use the patient's surname until corrected

Respectfully treat the patient as an equal

Don't Do This

Use a first name without permission

Mispronounce the name and not ask for help

Fail to make a note of correct pronunciation

Act arrogantly by ignoring the other's dignity

Fail to remember the name on a 2nd encounter

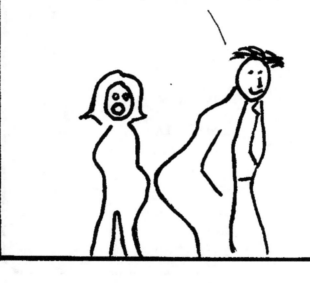

4

Handshakes and Other Greetings

IN THIS CHAPTER

Patients expect a culturally appropriate greeting but understand the importance of hand hygiene.

Nurses and other healthcare providers are encouraged to initiate the cultural shift to the "new normal" forms of greeting.

Doctors are reminded to explain the health reasons for not shaking hands and to model best practices encouraged by Departments of Public Health.

No one wants to blow a good first impression. And that means conforming with cultural non-verbal expectations. In polite society in North America when we greet one another and take our leave, it's the handshake. Elsewhere it may be "air kisses" on one or both cheeks, hugs, or other actions executed within one's "personal space." Failure to conform to the expected ritual typically raises eyebrows and produces muttering about rude "standoffishness."

So how does one deal with such tribal rites in the time of flu and pandemic? Healthcare workers should initiate the cultural change and model the behaviors encouraged by the Center for Disease Control and Departments of Public Health.[8] A number of new "future norms" have been suggested—a polite bow at the neck, arms folded across the chest, and fist or elbow bumps. But none of these will feel comfortable or friendly without practice and education.

---

[8] Center for Disease Control (CDC), "Keeping the workplace safe," 2019, https://www.cdc.gov/coronavirus/2019-ncov/downloads/workplace-school-and-home

It will be necessary for doctors and nurses to take the lead as they interact with patients. A patient health-centered explanation is recommended. For example, "It's a pleasure to meet you, Mr. Washington. Normally, I'd shake your hand but we are taking extra hygiene precautions to keep our patients safe. If you don't mind, I'll just give you a bow."

Most patients are familiar with the importance of hand hygiene and they understand the reason for improved safety measures. Chance the Rapper summed it up this way: "We only know what we know until someone knows better." With a patient-centered explanation, your encounter will likely be even more positive than if you had tried to shake hands or ignored the subject altogether.

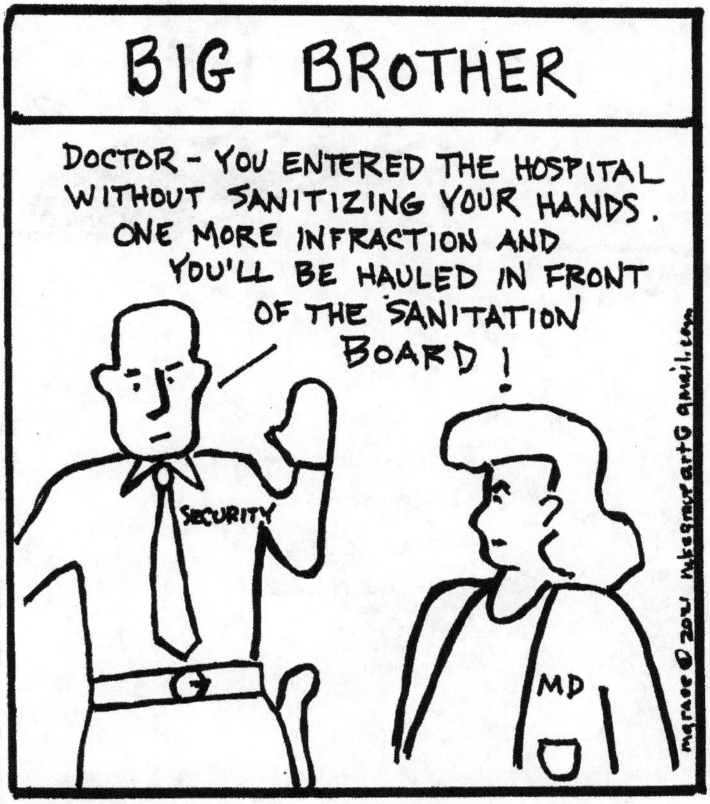
BIG BROTHER
DOCTOR - YOU ENTERED THE HOSPITAL WITHOUT SANITIZING YOUR HANDS. ONE MORE INFRACTION AND YOU'LL BE HAULED IN FRONT OF THE SANITATION BOARD!
SECURITY
MD

Do This

Model best healthcare hygiene practices

Initiate the cultural change in greetings

Offer a patient centered explanation for changes

Don't Do This

Continue to shake patients' hands

Ignore the new "cultural norms"

Ignore Dept of Public Health advice

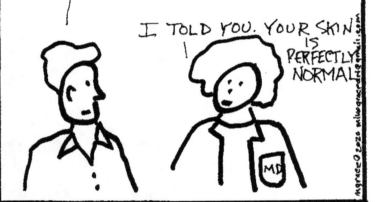

5

A Communication Model

IN THIS CHAPTER

Patients, nurses, and doctors are shown a simple communication model which emphasizes empathy in which Receivers use appropriate verbal and non-verbal feedback in response to any Sender's Message.

Whether your verbal exchange is a pre-operative doctor-patient meeting or a nurse's midnight phone call to a physician, the same communication dynamics are at play. Someone is saying something to another with the expectation the message will be understood as the sender intended. But too often, we know what is said has not been heard or understood in the same manner. And, unless the discrepancy is immediately recognized, subsequent comments only compound confusion and contribute to further conversational chaos. As playwright and author George Bernard Shaw wisely said: "The single biggest problem in communication is the illusion that it has taken place."

There are many communication models to illustrate the process. Let's take one of the most basic paradigms.[9] The Sender sends a Message to the Receiver who responds verbally or non-verbally in the form of Empathetic Feedback. Appropriate feedback fuels the sending of additional Messages. The lack of feedback or inappropriate feedback undermines the quality of the next Message. The roles of Sender and Receiver typically shift back and

---

[9] Gavi, Z., "The Models of Communication," The Communication Process, 2013 Aug 19, https://www.thecommunicationprocess.com/models-of-communication/

forth between the participants with Messages in the form of questions, answers or statements.

It's easier than it may sound. How many times have we been talking to a loved one and gotten no response. "Could you at least grunt to let me know you heard what I said!"

SENDER>>>>>MESSAGE>>>>>RECEIVER
<<<<<EMPATHETIC FEEDBACK<<<<<

The Empathetic Feedback can be non-verbal in the form of focused eye contact, an understanding nod, or a respectful hand pat. Non-interrupting verbal feedback can be in the form of the thoughtful "Um," the knowing "Uh huh," or the understanding "under the breath" "I see." And, of course, the next Message can be explicitly responsive and empathetic: "I understand what you're saying," "That must have been upsetting," "What happened next?" and so on. The key to Empathetic Feedback is the expression of compassionate understanding. It is what happens when we consciously try to walk in the shoes of another.

We all struggle to make ourselves understood, sometimes with great comedic effect. As comedian Groucho Marx related: "One morning I shot an elephant in my pajamas. How he got in my pajamas, I'll never know."

In future chapters we are going to apply this simple communication model to doctors, patients, and nurses. As we'll see, while many of the challenges for effective communication are universal to all human beings, some are quite unique to the participants in the healthcare setting. With enhanced awareness and armed with constructive strategies, every participant to the healthcare conversation will be able to improve their ability to send and receive Messages.

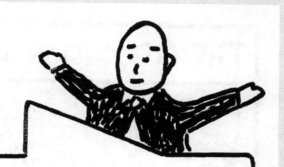

<u>Do This</u>

Be aware of the communication mode!

As Sender, speak clearly

As Receiver, listen actively

As Receiver, give Empathetic Feedback

<u>Don't Do This</u>

Assume the Message has been understood

Fail to assess verbal and non-verbal feedback

Refuse to try to see the other side

Fail to clarify the cause of misunderstandings

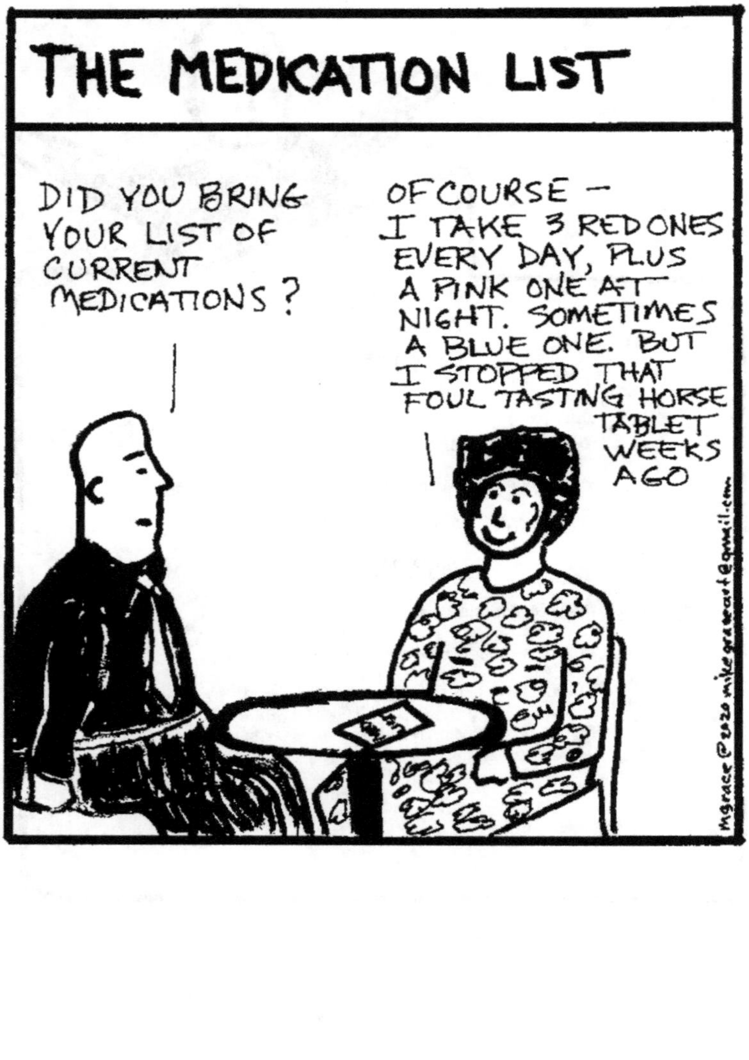
THE MEDICATION LIST
DID YOU BRING YOUR LIST OF CURRENT MEDICATIONS?
OF COURSE – I TAKE 3 RED ONES EVERY DAY, PLUS A PINK ONE AT NIGHT. SOMETIMES A BLUE ONE. BUT I STOPPED THAT FOUL TASTING HORSE TABLET WEEKS AGO
mgrace ©2020 mikegraceart@gmail.com

6
Interruption

IN THIS CHAPTER

Patients learn time pressures on healthcare providers, particularly doctors, may cause them to interrupt, even when the provider has asked for the patient's input.

Nurses are less prone to interrupt doctors or patients but doing so would have the same deleterious impact on effective communication.

Doctors who interrupt undermine their own communication efforts which may hinder accurate diagnosis and treatment and, if constant, may damage the professional relationship.

Almost everyone bemoans the fast pace of their life. But for healthcare professionals it can be pressure on steroids. It is not always possible to take actor Lily Tomlin's clever advice: "For fast acting relief, try slowing down."

Where else is there a greater expectation of perfect job performance each and every day? What other industry is as highly regulated with so many judgmental eyes watching for a slip-up? How many other professions face true life and death decisions? Add to the mix staff shortages, medical emergencies, and public health crises and it's no wonder doctors and nurses feel extraordinary pressures to get everything done accurately, perfectly, and quickly.

And this perceived "need for speed" leads to one of the greatest, but most easily corrected communication problems of them all—interrupting the speaker. Numerous academic studies have examined the issue. Shockingly, the majority of physicians interrupt their patients after only 11 seconds![10] Male physicians tend to do so more than female physicians but both male and female doctors interrupt woman patients more than men. Even when asked to tell their story, sadly patients are commonly and quickly interrupted.

There are many expected consequences of these interruptions. The communication process becomes derailed. Trains of thought are lost. Messages are garbled. Important information may be overlooked or omitted affecting accurate diagnosis and treatment. Understandably patients become irritated. Constant interruption may lead to serious damage to the relationship. Ironically, interrupting the patient may not even achieve the goal of saving time as thoughts must be refocused or arguments ensue.

There are no studies of interruptions by patients or nurses, probably because they occur less frequently. But logically one would expect a patient or nurse interrupting a physician would have all the same potential ill effects.

Healthcare providers, especially doctors, need to practice self-restraint. Bite your tongue if necessary, especially during the first few minutes of the patient encounter. Old habits die hard. If you slip up and interrupt, quickly apologize and allow the patient to continue. The courtesy will be appreciated and the ground rules established. The patient will be more likely to follow your example of uninterrupted listening.

---

[10] Phillips, K., Ospina, N., Montori, V., "Physicians Interrupting Patients," Journal of General Internal Medicine, 2019 Oct; 34(10): 1965

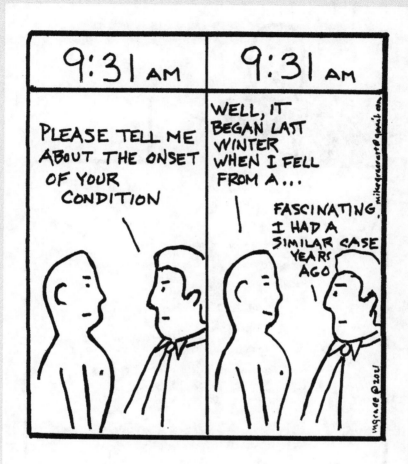

Do This

Slow down and listen especially at the outset

Be aware of gender biased interruptions

Give yourself the chance to hear about priorities

Apologize if you interrupt

Don't Do This

Ignore patient concerns and priorities

Rush to correct the patient

Treat female patients differently than males

Let interruptions distract from the Message

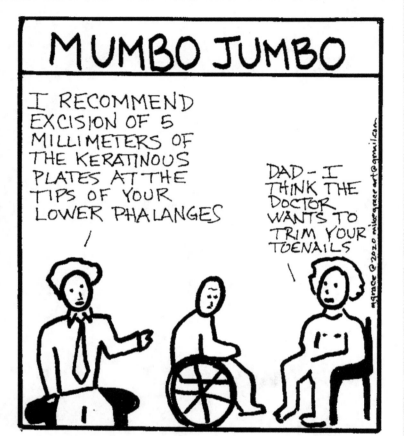

7

Technical Talk

IN THIS CHAPTER

Patients learn a major barrier to understanding medical information from their healthcare providers--doctors and nurses--is the failure to speak plainly.

Nurses and doctors are shown how to take the mumbo jumbo out of their speech by using best communication practices.

The heart of most doctor-patient-nurse interactions is the communication of medically pertinent and often technical information. This can be challenging because only 12% of U.S. adults are highly proficient when it comes to understanding health information.[11] How should the doctor or nurse communicate complex concepts without confusing or turning off the patient? It's not hard. It just takes a conscious effort and some practice. In a nutshell, talk to your patient like you'd talk to your own mom or dad about what you do. Speak plainly and try not to convolute it. As British prime minister and writer Winston Churchill admonished: "This is the sort of English up with which I will not put."

Unfortunately, many healthcare providers, particularly doctors, when speaking to patients slip into comfortable professional language better reserved for their colleagues. Here is a true story of my own family's experience:

We knew it was the day of reckoning. Our first meeting with the doctor who would disclose the treatment for my father's diagnosed lung cancer. The medical assistant shepherded my mom, dad, and me into the surgeon's private office. He was already there, sheltered behind his impressive desk, face back-lit

---

[11] Killian, L., Coletti, M., "The role of universal health literacy precautions in minimizing 'medspeak' and promoting shared decision making," AMA J Ethics, 2017; 19(3): 296–303

by the partially drawn shades blocking the late afternoon sun. We took our seats, mom and I flanking dad facing the doctor across the room.

The doctor greeted us with a smile but remained seated. "Good afternoon. Thank you for being on time." There were no introductions. I tried to discern from his expression what was to come and replied: "Of course. We've been anxiously waiting for today." My parents merely nodded in agreement, having been too shocked to say much the past couple of days.

The doctor continued: "I want you to know I have reviewed all of the imaging studies as well as the accompanying radiology reports, reviewed the pathology findings from the biopsy, and personally spoken with both the radiologist and pathologist. My partners and I have also briefly conferred about your case. We are all in agreement that due to the size and location of the tumor adjacent to the bronchus in the upper chest, your lesion is not resectable."

He paused and waited for the news to sink in. As a medical malpractice trial attorney who'd handled many cancer cases, I struggled for the meaning. My mind raced. Resectable? Somewhere I'd previously heard the term. As in "resection"? As in "not capable of resection"? Oh my God. Now, for a brief moment, two people in the room knew what was happening.

My dad turned to me. "What's he saying, Mike?" I took a deep breath. "Dad, I think the doctor just said your lung cancer is inoperable; it can't be removed by surgery." My father looked away trying to absorb the news while my mother fought back tears.

"Yes, Mr. Grace. I'm afraid what your son indicated is correct. However, there are other viable treatment options including adjuvant chemotherapy and radiation for both the primary lesion and the metastatic disease. I've already taken the liberty of setting up appointments for you to be seen by our oncologists." The meeting quickly ended with the doctor's expression of regret.

Shortly thereafter, we met with the radiation and medication cancer specialists and my dad agreed to their recommended treatment plan. He underwent the therapy but passed away from his disease seven months later.

My family's experience is not unique. This type of verbal interaction between healthcare provider and patient happens every day. Confusing mumbo jumbo which fails to communicate effectively.

Here is how to take the mumbo jumbo out of your speech:

• Avoid all unnecessary medical jargon. Most patients will understand "not operable" better than "not resectable." The "spread of cancer to other organs" is clearer than "metastatic disease." "Adjuvant chemotherapy?" How about saying "chemo" instead? Remember, the goal is not to impress the patient with how erudite you are, but to speak clearly.

- Define medical terms as soon as they are used. It is appropriate to use medical words in a medical conversation, just immediately clarify the meaning of necessary medical terms. "Oncology" is a recognized medical specialty but most people will better comprehend "cancer radiation specialist" than "radiation oncologist."

- Use analogies and common references whenever possible. For example, orthopedic surgery is often compared to carpentry; cardiac and urinary surgery to plumbing.

- Use pictures and diagrams to illustrate. Creating your own simplified drawings with the patient watching allows you slowly to explain. This is usually more effective than using intricate professional anatomical illustrations. For example: "Your primary tumor is located here where I've drawn the top of the right lung near these bronchial airways."

- Use academic doctor-oriented literature sparingly. Remember most American adults read at only a grade school level. However, there is an abundance of material geared to the general patient population such as brochures created by professional societies and academies.

- Speak respectfully on an adult level but this seldom requires more than three syllable words.

- But never talk down to a patient. You should be striving to hit the sweet spot found by medical experts in court when explaining medical concepts to lay jurors.

- Encourage questions, carefully listening to the feedback for clues of what needs to be clarified or restated. The Sender must constantly be observing the Receiver "audience."

- Ask the patient to restate in his own words what he has been told to do. This feedback loop, also known as "teach-back," ensures the Receiver accurately understood the Sender's Message. Of course, patients should never hesitate to speak up if they have any doubt about what the healthcare provider has said. The medical professional may have misread your look of confusion.

- Remain calm and remember you are the expert while the patient is just now trying to master a slice of your knowledge.

- Remember most of us need to hear a message three times before it's been fully absorbed. There's a reason you learned in high school and college speech classes always to use an introduction, body, and conclusion—tell them what you are going to tell them, tell them, and tell them what you told them.

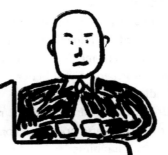

Do This

Talk plainly without medical jargon

Explain all necessary medical terms

Make your own drawings to explain a concept

Be respectful and patient with your listener

Encourage questions to verify understanding

Don't Do This

Use mumbo jumbo and convoluted speech

Use academic literature or complex drawings

Talk down to a patient

Fail to "read your audience" for comprehension

Fail to patiently answer questions

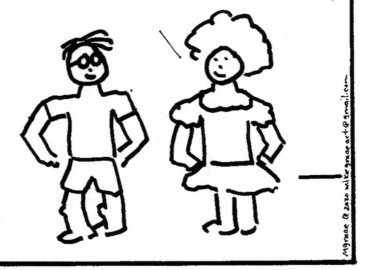

8
Patient Barriers to Understanding

IN THIS CHAPTER

Patients learn there are many obstacles to understanding a healthcare provider's Message including their own biases and health illiteracy among other barriers.

Nurses and doctors are shown strategies for overcoming the barriers including awareness, demonstration of competence and trustworthiness, as well as projection of a friendly, non-threatening demeanor.

Even in a perfect world where the doctor conveys a clear message with professional decorum, there is often a forest of undergrowth blocking and distorting the Message from being received as the doctor intended. The doctor righteously believes "I did my job! Why didn't the patient listen or speak up?" Meanwhile, the patient is prepared to swear under oath "He never told me a thing!"

The potential obstacles experienced by the patient are manifold:

- Bias. This can be against the Sender healthcare professional, the Sender's profession, or the Message itself. Bias is often attached to the Receiver's core beliefs which can be difficult to dislodge. For example, there may be ethnic prejudice against Muslims, distrust of chiropractic medicine, or suspicion of childhood vaccinations. The best strategy is to dazzle the patient with a display of competence and trustworthiness discussed in Chapter 14.

- Health illiteracy. This is defined by the American Medical Association as a "constellation of skills, including the ability to perform basic reading and numerical tasks required to function in the health care environment." In 2004, the Institute of Medicine estimated 90 million adults have trouble understanding and acting on health information. Two provider strategies are required: First, recognizing patient behaviors suggestive of inadequate health literacy skills such as asking for help, bringing along someone who can read, inability to keep appointments, making excuses, medication non-compliance, poor adherence to the treatment plans, postponing decision making, and mimicking the behavior of others. Second, once recognized, providers need to take steps to enhance understanding such as slowing down, using simpler language, drawing pictures, limiting information given at each encounter, and using "teach back" to confirm patient understanding, all done with a caring and respectful attitude.[12]
- White coat stress. This phenomenon actually increases vital signs and impairs the patient's ability to receive the Sender's Message as intended. Be aware of your patient's emotional state and become the affable approachable doctor also profiled in Chapter 14.
- Pain. Physical discomfort blocks all lesser demanding stimuli such as a nurse's explanation and instruction. Read your patient's body language. It may be time for an analgesic before meaningful dialogue is possible.
- Medication. The effects of medication, individually or in combination with one another, can affect everything from cognition to personality. Constant vigilance is required, especially when the patient is receiving medication from multiple doctors.
- Memory impairment. This has many causes but is a natural part of the aging process especially short-term memory loss among the elderly.
- Sensory loss. This too has many causes ranging from medication to illness and can affect hearing, speech and motor skills.
- Language barriers. Non-English speakers, no matter how proficient with common chit chat, may lack the linguistic tools to understand a medical vocabulary.
- Cultural confusion. Foreign born patients may not understand their new surroundings or know how to read cultural cues.

---

[12] Safeer, R., Keenan, J., "Health Literacy: The Gap Between Physicians and Patients," Am Fam Physician, 2005 Aug 1; 72(3): 463–468

- Fear of treatment. Fear is a primal emotion which triggers "fight or flight." Fear of the medical unknown is common. Worry about the ability to work or function with medical treatment can drown out a Sender's reassuring Message.
- Terror of death and dying. Many of us, especially the young, glide through life with a false sense of immortality until we hit the inevitable wall. The shock can block all healthcare Messages.

Some of these situations are deserving of special attention—such as communicating with the elderly (chapter 31), foreign language speakers (chapter 24), and the seriously ill (chapter 32).

In every encounter it is incumbent on the provider to assess for potential barriers to patient understanding and tailor her Message accordingly. For example, the doctor always needs to begin a visit with a reconciliation of the patient's medications with an eye to potential effects on cognition, memory, and motor skills.[13] Does the patient appear alert, tired, or unsteady? In other words, always "read" the audience you are speaking to. And then act accordingly.

And the provider needs to be aware of the competing stimuli to her own Message. These are typically non-medical in nature and affect the Sender and Receiver equally. Is the room too hot or too cold? Is there distracting noise emanating from the hallway or public address system? Is it the lunch hour and are stomachs rumbling? The types of distractions are potentially infinite, some outside the Sender's control, but all must be taken into account.

---

[13] The Joint Commission, "Ambulatory Health Care National Patient Safety Goals, NPSG.03.06.01," 2020

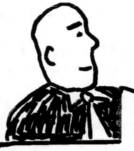

Do This

Counter bias with confidence and trustworthiness

Counter white coat stress with friendliness

Read patient body language for signs of pain

Look for physical/mental effects of medication

Be sensitive to fears of treatment and death

Don't Do This

Overlook strategies to overcome the barriers

Ignore deeply held patient biases

Fail to reconcile medications every visit

Be insensitive to language/cultural differences

Ignore non-medical barriers to understanding

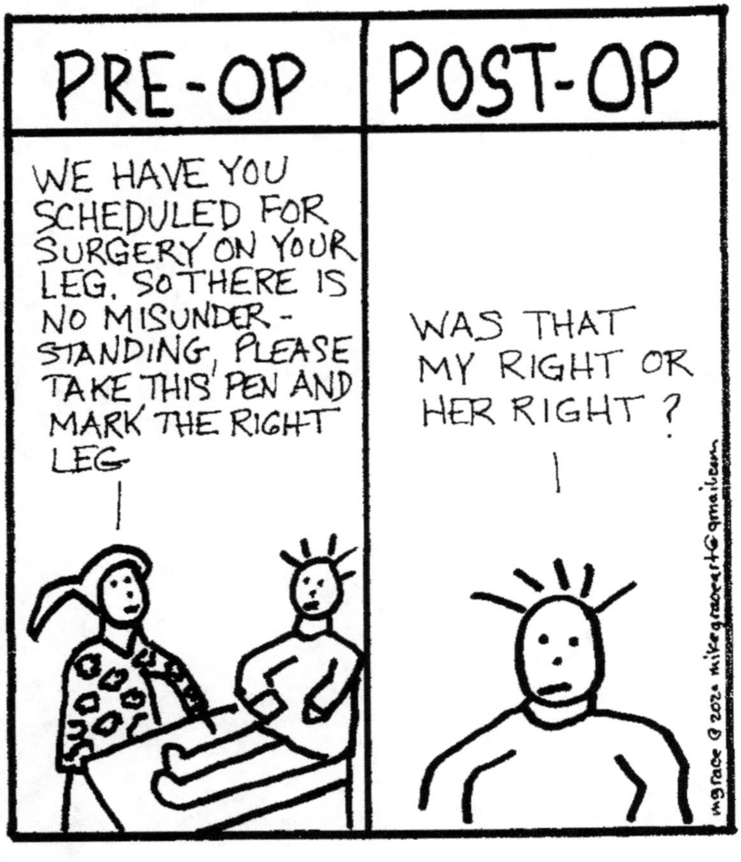
PRE-OP
POST-OP
WE HAVE YOU SCHEDULED FOR SURGERY ON YOUR LEG. SO THERE IS NO MISUNDER-STANDING, PLEASE TAKE THIS PEN AND MARK THE RIGHT LEG
WAS THAT MY RIGHT OR HER RIGHT ?

9
It's More About Listening

IN THIS CHAPTER

Patients, nurses and doctors discover active listening by the Receiver is the key to effective communication which occurs when all the participants are fully engaged in the interactive process. They learn to read the clues to unpack the Sender's Message and strategies how to decipher the meaning behind the words.

The common fallacy when discussing communication skills is that it's mostly about talking. In truth, it's more about listening.[14] Not just hearing (although functioning tympanic membranes are useful!), but actively concentrating on the words being spoken and the meaning behind the words. Most of us have probably thought what comic Margaret Cho dared to say: "I want Jesus to come back and say 'THAT'S NOT WHAT I MEANT.'"

Active listening is actually more exhausting than talking. It is only by active listening the Receiver truly experiences the Message as intended by the Sender. Fortunately, neither the provider nor the patient needs to be a mind reader. The clues are literally in front of us. To become successful active listeners (Receivers of Messages), we just need to learn how to decipher them.

Here are the important clues:

- Does the Message seem clear on its face?
- Is the Sender's body language congruent with the Message?

---

[14] Tayal, S., Michelson, K., Tayal, N., "Empathetic Listening," AMA STEPS Forward, 2016 Aug 31, https://www.edhub.ama-assn.org/steps-forward/module/2702561

- Is the Sender's tone of voice in sync with the words spoken?
- Is the Message consistent with prior Messages?
- Is the Message believable?
- Is a surprisingly unbelievable Message due to the patient spinning a tale for the benefit of a family member in the room? Or does the Message of the healthcare provider make an unfounded assumption about the patient's medical condition?
- Is the Sender credible?

If any "red flags" are raised by any of these questions, here are some suggested next steps:

- Ask open-ended questions for clarification. "What do you mean?" "How often did that happen?" "How did you form that opinion?" Non-open-ended questions are best left to the lawyer's courtroom cross examination. Those are the questions which suggest the answer. "Isn't it true at the last office visit you told me you never experience sleeplessness?" Remember, your goal should be to obtain information which clarifies the meaning behind the words, not engage in a game of "gotcha."
- Keep asking "why?" This is the fundamental technique used by hospital risk managers when conducting a root cause analysis of an adverse event. The technique is well suited to finding the real reason why something happened rather than merely accepting the "official" or "initial" explanation. For example, a patient may state he didn't take his medication. Repeatedly asking "why" could lead to the following answers: "I often run out." "I often run out because I don't like to take it." "I don't like to take it because it upsets my stomach."
- Gently suggest the patient's words seem to be at odds with the non-verbal message. For example, the patient denies being depressed—but her affect is flat and her arms are defensively crossed over her chest. You might say: "Mrs. Chu, I'm pleased to hear you say so, but you don't seem your normal cheerful self today. Is anything bothering you?"

Active listening occurs when the Receiver is truly engaged in the interpersonal process. It is characterized by appropriate verbal and non-verbal Empathetic Feedback in the communication model. Active listening is demonstrated by paying attention, leaning in while focusing on the speaker, and maintaining an open body posture. This is in contrast with passive listening typically characterized by a lack of feedback. Often the passive listener is thinking more about what he is going to say next than concentrating on the Sender's Message. And passive listeners are often easily distracted by the bombardment of competing stimuli—intrusive thoughts of what they'll do later at home, the smell of the other person's aftershave or perfume, the buzz of the fly on the window, to name a few.

And, of course, active listening is antithetical to the Receiver who insists on usurping the role of Sender. This occurs by constantly interrupting, hogging the conversation, raising irrelevant off-topic subjects, and using any comment by the Sender as another opportunity to discuss themselves. As the self-absorbed actress played by Bette Midler in the movie "Beaches" says to her girlfriend after a lengthy personal monologue: "Enough about me...Let's talk about you. What do you think about me?" Healthcare should not be about the provider; it should always be focused on the patient.

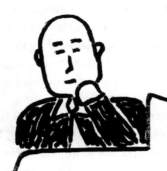

Do This

Actively listen

Put yourself in the shoes of the other person

Listen for the meaning behind the words

Look for clues of body language and tone of voice

Ask open-ended and "why" questions for insight

Don't Do This

Be a passive listener

Ignore inconsistent behavior by the Sender

Fail to question inconsistent Messages

Think about what you're going to say next

Give no feedback or inappropriate feedback

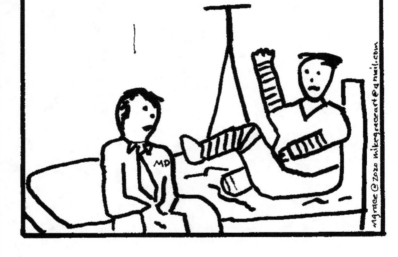

10
Human Barriers
to Active Listening

IN THIS CHAPTER

Patients, nurses, and doctors learn how body language, body position, and tone of voice impact their Messages.

Doctors learn that standing when speaking to a seated or reclining patient impedes the effectiveness of their Message.

Apart from medical and non-medical obstacles to active listening, there are actual human barriers which prevent the Sender's Message from being heard by the Receiver as intended. Any one of them can impede access to the full attention of the Receiver; in combination they can become an impregnable fortress. Some of the most impactful are non-verbal body language, body positioning, and tone of voice.

The Sender's body language says more than his words. Screen legend Mae West reminded us: "I speak two languages. Body and English." Tense body language—fists clenched for example—give lie to a verbal message of soothing comfort. Nervous laughter undercuts the truth of a message of reassurance. Not surprisingly, most communication studies confirm more information is intuited by non-verbal signals than understood by explicit verbal expression. Moreover, the non-verbal language is usually found to be much more believable than the spoken word.[15] How often have we heard ourselves say, "I just don't trust him. He looks shifty." "She seems so insincere always flashing that phony smile." Let's face it. No matter how much someone says, "You can trust me," if we're not seeing it and feeling it, we are not believing it!

Therefore, the Sender must constantly be mindful of a congruence between her verbal and non-verbal communication. The lack of such consistency is called dissonance. While we all may not be familiar with the term, we all know the experience. Hence the expression: "We don't always remember what a person says, but we always remember how they made us feel."

One's physical body position can also be a human barrier to active listening. A doctor who stands over a patient is impeding his own message. Not only is it discourteous and domineering, but physically uncomfortable for the patient to strain looking up. Studies from a large Midwestern hospital confirm the standing provider is perceived by the patient as being impatient and has somewhere else to go. The doctor who sits is perceived as more caring than one who stands. Patients also report a more positive interaction and a better understanding of their condition.[16]

And interestingly, even if the sitting doctor spends less time than the standing physician, the patient perceives more time has been spent with the sitting doctor. Physicians and patients who feel time pressure, especially during the brief appointment allotted for a focused office visit, should take note. Doctors should always remain seated—your limited time will appear stretched in the eyes of the patient.

While sitting on the same level as the patient is a positive, the provider should never sit on the patient's bed. Most patients perceive this an invasion of their personal space. Jostling of the bed can also be painful to the patient. He's in bed for a reason! The practice is also unhygienic. Pull up a chair at bedside and have your talk.

Finally, tone of voice is just as important as non-verbal body language and body position. No one processes information well when they are being yelled at. Raised voices simply are not effective Message transmitters. Paradoxically, attention increases when the voice is lowered, not when it is raised. Stage actors have known this secret for millennia. The lowered voice instinctively

---

[15] Mager, D., "The 4 Primary Principles of Communication," Psychology Today, 2007 Feb 13, https://www.psychologytoday.com/us/blog/some-assembly-required201702/the-4-primary-principles-communication

[16] Swayden, K., Anderson, K., et al., "Effect of sitting vs. standing on perception of provider time at bedside: a pilot study," Patient Educ Couns, 2012 Feb; 86(2): 166–171

causes the listener to pay closer attention. Sarcastic and sneering tones are as off-putting—and insulting—as the raised voice.

Unfortunately, in the world of healthcare with its truly life and death dramas, too often providers (mostly male physicians) attempt to excuse bullying insults and screaming tantrums as a necessary evil of the work culture. As a hospital Chief-of-Staff once told me, "Those nurses just need to pull on their 'big girl pants' and deal with it." Well, as the Risk Manager replied: "No one needs to be demeaned or harassed on the job. It's called a hostile work environment and if unchecked will likely lead to a lawsuit."

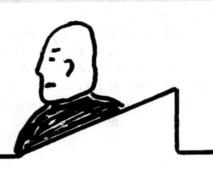

Do This

Read body language for meaning

Listen to tone of voice for meaning

Consider body positioning when speaking

Make verbal and non-verbal messages consistent

Sit on the same level to project a caring attitude

Don't Do This

Ignore feelings about the Sender or Message

Ignore conflicting verbal and non-verbal clues

Stand over your seated patient

Sit on the patient's bed

Yell or use sarcasm in professional speech

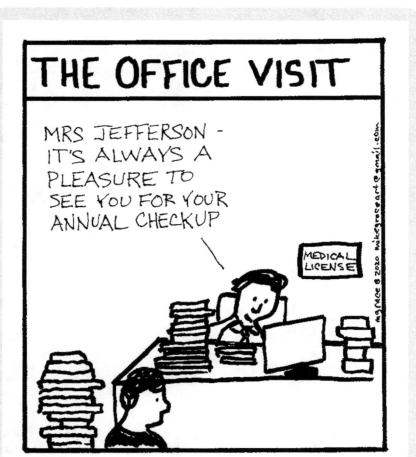

11
Physical Barriers to Active Listening

IN THIS CHAPTER

Patients recognize physical impediments to a satisfactory conversation with their healthcare providers.

Nurses and doctors are reminded all professional conversations should be conducted in private places free from physical distractions.

Even something as mundane as a medical office set-up can sabotage excellent communication and impair the Receiver's ability to process the Sender's Message. Here are some common problems posed by physical barriers:

- Corner computer placement in exam rooms. The prevalence of electronic medical records makes the computer an essential tool. But putting it in the corner requires the operator's back to be toward the room and the provider not facing the patient. Again, this interferes with the free flow of communication. But even more importantly, its corner placement says "the computer monitor is my priority, not you." One can already hear the disgruntled patient: "The doctor virtually ignored me during the examination. All I saw was the back of his head. He just stared at that damned computer screen!"[17]

---

[17] Gaffey, A., Groves, S., "The Clinical Record," In Carroll, R., (ed), *Risk Management Handbook for Healthcare Organizations*, 6th edition, 2011; 331, 355

- Office furniture. Some doctors still hide behind their mahogany desks. Intended or not, the non-verbal message is a relationship of inequality and authority. It enforces separation and reinforces a false sense of superiority. Of course, this is seldom considered or intended by the desk's proud owner. It may be a family heirloom but the perceived message is unflattering. The same message is also conveyed by the contrast between the doctor's high-backed executive chair and the low-backed smaller client chair. Of course, doctors aren't the only offenders; we lawyers have been guilty of this set-up for years!
- The best practice is a small bare table with equally sized chairs where provider and patient are speaking on the same level with unobstructed views of the other. A computer stand on wheels can be moved out of the way but still accessed if reading or making electronic notes are critical during the meeting. Better than a large computer monitor is a less obtrusive electronic tablet.
- Messy desks. Desks piled high with books, journals, and computer monitors obstruct a clear sight line between the parties. Not only is it rude and unin-viting, but it impairs the ability to read each other's body language. Most people with messy work environments insist they know where everything is located. While this might occasionally be true, the non-verbal message is mental sloppiness and disarray. When a lawsuit is filed alleging the doctor negligently forgot to do something, one can already hear the patient's testimony: "It's no wonder he forgot—he is so disorganized. You wouldn't believe what a disaster his desk is!"
- Cell phones. Most healthcare environments post signs discouraging cell phone use. Cell phones should be silenced by all participants during the encounter. When a patient takes a call while meeting with a physician or nurse, his action sends a strong non-verbal message of disrespect. When the provider takes a call "on the patient's time" irritation and resentment are likely. If the provider is using his smart phone to research a quick point pertinent to the discussion, tell the patient what you are doing to avoid any misunderstanding. "I just want to refresh my recollection about whether weight gain has been reported by the drug manufacturer as a potential side effect."
- Music systems. No matter how soothing the provider finds her taste in music, playing the radio, stereo, or a personal cell phone playlist is annoying and disruptive when meeting with others. Popular lyrics tug on memories and even instrumentals invite tapping a beat. Turning the music down is no

solution; the human brain will instinctively strain to hear. It all divides the attention of our minds. Save the music for private office time even if you and your patient share the same musical tastes.

- Exposed examination spaces. Exam spaces which lack complete privacy will bother most patients. Undrawn curtains or visible sight lines from opened doors will distract many patients from giving the provider's Message their full attention. Patients are always within their rights to insist their dignity and privacy be respected.

- Hallways. All healthcare communication must be private. Selecting a public venue like a hallway to talk to a patient or nurse is guaranteed to create problems. Passersby become distractions and perhaps an unintended audience. Public locations encourage grandstanding and emotional conflict. Always find a private place for private conversations.

- Too often doctors choose to speak to the nurse where others can hear. Not a huge problem if the doctor is lavishing the nurse with praise. But more often it is an occasion for a public and embarrassing reprimand of perceived shortcomings. Likewise, nurses should also select a non-public space to air grievances to a physician. And do so in a calm, quiet, and respectful tone. Anything less poisons the well of professional discourse.

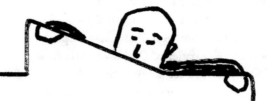

Do This

Face your patient on the same physical level

Keep your environment as organized as your mind

Explain any necessary use of your cell phone

Ensure examination spaces are private

Have private conversations in private places

Don't Do This

Hide behind your computer monitor

Keep your back to the patient

Sit behind your big desk

Play music during exams or meetings

Speak about private matters in hallways

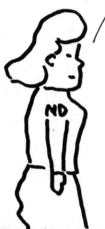
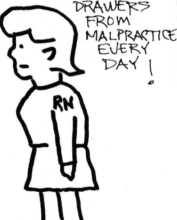

12

Nurse-Doctor Communication

IN THIS CHAPTER

Patients discover there is too often a tension between their doctors and nurses which negatively impacts patient care.

Nurses are given strategies to improve their relationships with physicians and are encouraged to use SBAR as a standard tool for face-to-face and telephonic communications.

Doctors learn reasons why relationships with nurses are often not as positive as they imagine and how to improve communication including waiting for the nurse's accurate read-back of orders.

Historically there has been a tension between nurses and doctors stemming from outmoded notions of job hierarchy, gender roles, and differences of education and class. Fortunately, the situation has improved considerably, especially in areas like the OR and ICU which emphasize a team approach to patient care. While nurse-doctor relations are better within collaborative groups, bias and bad behavior persist in other areas of healthcare, especially among some older physicians. A large 2013 survey reported almost one-third of respondents believed there were "too many unprofessional clashes" between nurses and doctors.[18]

The problem is particularly vexing because of the disparity in perceptions between many doctors and nurses about the quality of their relationships.

---

[18] Jessie, C., "How To Build a Better Doctor Nurse Relationship," Med Study, 2020 May 6, https.//www.mkt.medstudy.com/glog/how-to-build-better-doctor-nurse-relationship

Doctors tend to think the relationships are significantly better than nurses rate the same relationships. Doctors often don't see the same lack of trust and respect felt by many nurses.[19]

The impact on patient safety, career satisfaction, and employee retention is real. All have been well documented and come as no real surprise. Who stays in a job without trust or respect? Who rushes to interact with someone known to be disagreeable? For example, in one study, 55% of nurses admitted a physician's behavior impacted nursing decisions. They are less quick to contact a "problem" doctor. Younger, less experienced nurses in particular, are more affected than their older peers by negative physician behavior.[20]

Many of the incidents I investigated as a hospital Risk Manager were triggered by the complaint of a patient who overheard an unprofessional exchange between doctor and nurse. Witnessing such behavior not only upsets patients, but more importantly undermines their confidence in the care they are receiving.

As with most communication relationships, solutions are never one-sided. Empathizing with the other person usually sheds light on ways to improve. Here are some suggestions for doctors:

- Use the nurse's name. Just like patients, everyone wants to feel acknowledged and recognized.
- Show respect for the nurse-patient relationship. They spend a lot more time together and probably have a rapport you may not have established. Doctors should keep in mind nurses are consistently held in the highest esteem of any professional group. In both the 2012 and 2019 Gallup surveys, nurses were viewed by 85% of respondents as highly or very highly regarded. Physicians have dropped 20 points lower and we lawyers are barely above used car salesmen at 22%.[21]
- Create a culture of inclusion. Discuss the care plan, especially on complicated cases.
- As with good patient communication, actively listen without interrupting.

---

[19] Siediecki, S., Hixson, E., "Relationships Between Nurses and Physicians Matter," The Online Journal of Issues in Nursing, 2015 Aug 31; 20(3)

[20] Benner, A., "Physician and nurse relationships, a key to patient safety," J Ky Med Assoc, 2007: 105(4): 165–169

[21] Gallup Politics, "Nurses Again Outpace Other Professions for Honesty, Ethics," 2018 Dec 20, https.//www.news.gallup.com/pdf/245597/nurses-again-outpace

- Don't be a rude bully on the telephone by saying things you'd probably not dare say face-to-face. No matter how late the hour or unfocused the nurse's comments.
- If you've acted badly, raised your voice, or used a disparaging tone, apologize. Sincerely and without delay.

Here are what nurses can do to improve the relationship:

- Respect the doctor's time and get to the point. Take a page from the military's playbook by remembering BLUF—bottom line up front. Know the facts and be organized in your thoughts. Don't apologize for "bothering him." If you understand why you are calling, you are both just doing your jobs. If you are unsure why you want to call, first discuss the patient's condition with your nursing chain of command for more experienced guidance about how to proceed.
- Always be respectful and professional, even if the doctor does not respond in kind. But be direct in calling out unacceptable behavior, especially if it persists. "Doctor, there is no reason to raise your voice. I can hear you perfectly well."
- Keep your private conversations private. Don't complain to other staff members about the doctor. Save reports of inappropriate doctor encounters for your supervisor.
- Give the doctor the benefit of the doubt. Don't presume the worst intention and don't jump on every perceived shortcoming. Doctors are under considerable stress and time pressure. Some bruised feelings are inevitable. Just keep it in perspective. And try to keep your sense of humor.
- Take the time to acknowledge and thank the doctor who responded to your request. Yes, she was just doing her job, but we all like to feel appreciated.

We know there are many reasons for doctors and nurses to misunderstand each another. One reason is the lack of similar communication skills training. In 2006, The Joint Commission recommended a standardized communication tool, SBAR, to be used between healthcare providers.[22] The goal was "to promote good communication and teamwork and to prevent errors and

---

[22] Shaneela, S., Sumesh, T., "Situation, Background, Assessment, Recommendation (SBAR) Communication Tool for Handoff in Health Care-A Narrative Review," Safety in Health, 2018, 4(7): 2–5

improve patient outcomes." It has been successfully adopted by most nursing programs. Unfortunately, most physicians are still unaware of it—unless they've recently graduated from medical school or work in an integrated healthcare delivery system which employs them and can enforce "standardized" procedures.

SBAR is a straightforward simple construct to organize verbal nurse-doctor exchanges whether telephonic or face-to-face.

S=Situation. Identify yourself and the current situation, observations and concerns.

"This is Nurse Steven Block calling from 2 East at Memorial Hospital about your patient, Ms. Coleman in Room 2104—I'm concerned she may have a lung infection. She is complaining of shortness of breath, worsening with exertion. Her oxygen saturation was 88%. She was placed on 2 liters of oxygen and her O2 sat is now 90%. Her respirations are 26, pulse 108, blood pressure 94/62, temperature is 102. She has a productive cough with bloody mucous and reports pain when coughing on a scale of 9 out of 10."

B=Background.

"Ms. Coleman has a history of COPD for 5 years. On admission she had a cough and was diagnosed with a COPD exacerbation. She was prescribed a bronchodilator every 4 hours."

A=Assessment.

"I think the patient is exhibiting symptoms which may be associated with pneumonia."

R=Recommendation.

Would you like me to obtain a stat x-ray? Should I start an IV for antibiotics?" "Will you be coming in to see the patient?

Consistent use of SBAR offers mutual advantages to both parties. It requires the nurse to be prepared for the physician interaction. He must be knowledgeable about the patient's history, signs, symptoms, current treatment, and change in condition. And it focuses the nurse's attention before the interaction on what he hopes to get from the doctor. A physician familiar with SBAR knows at the outset what to expect and, if necessary, can prompt the nurse to return to the format. Both sides have a road map where they are going and will know when they have arrived.

However, the use of SBAR alone will not solve the nurse-doctor communication problem if the impatient doctor is resistant to the nurse reading back the orders. Many pharmaceutical names sound similar and it is easy to misunderstand or mishear numeric dosage and administration time intervals like the antibiotic IV infusion in our SBAR example. This is a chronic problem with foreign born doctors with thick accents, and it often occurs during calls in the middle of the night. Best patient safety practice is for the doctor always to stay on the line until the nurse accurately reads back all of the orders.

As they say, success breeds success. With each positive nurse-doctor interaction the odds increase the next one will also be smoother and more satisfying.

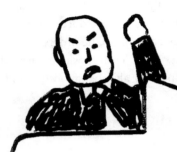

Do This

Use SBAR in doctor-nurse communication

Respect each other's special expertise

Create a culture of inclusion

Know your facts and what you want

Apologize if communication gets heated

Don't Do This

Gossip to staff about run-ins

Presume a bad intention on the other side

Bully or shame the other person

Hang up before the order's read-back

Forget to thank each other

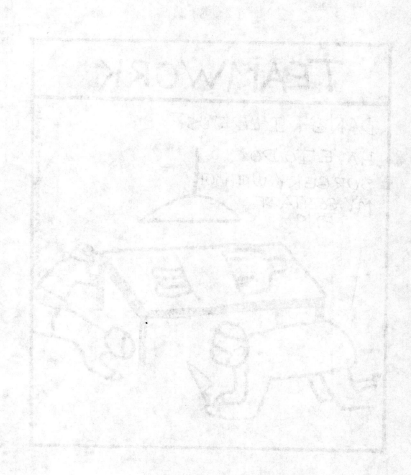

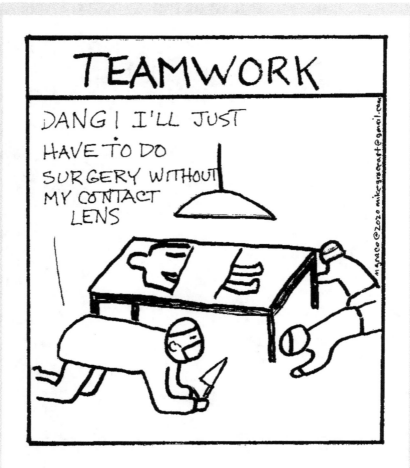

13
Communication Within Teams

IN THIS CHAPTER

Patients learn standardized safety communication protocols among healthcare providers are sometimes omitted which increases the risk of medical errors.

Nurses are urged to speak up when they see standardized protocols being ignored.

Doctors and nurses are encouraged to recognize time pressures can result in unsafe shortcuts.

Team building is a popular trend in healthcare. It promotes cooperation, trust and respect, improves communication and enhances patient outcomes. Most of the time.

But the camaraderie and familiarity of working with the same group of people can carry unappreciated risk to patient safety—a breakdown of standardized communication protocols based on a misplaced trust in one another. Working daily with the same team of highly trained colleagues both impresses and lulls us into letting down our guard and skipping steps in defined processes. In the world of risk assessment and mitigation, this phenomenon is known as a human risk factor.

Standardized healthcare procedures took their inspiration from the disciplined field of aeronautics.[23] Cockpit protocols are step specific behaviors

---

[23] Roberts, K., Yu, K., van Stralen, D., "Patient safety is an organizational systems issue: lessons from a variety of industries." In Youngberg, B. and Hatlie, M. (eds.) *The Patient Safety Handbook*, Canada: Jones and Bartlett, 2004

written in checklist form and audibly confirmed by another team member. No matter how many flight hours a pilot and co-pilot have logged together, each and every time they prepare to take-off or land they methodically perform the required drill. Without exception. Who among us would feel safe flying on a plane if we were told the cockpit opted to skip the checklist that day?

The "time-out" universal protocols in operating rooms are a good example of the use of required checklist behaviors. No surgery should commence without first taking the time to confirm out loud in the presence of the entire OR team the identity of the patient, the nature of the surgery, and the specific surgical site. And it works almost all the time—unless the OR is running behind schedule and the surgeon tries to skip the "time-out." It takes a strong and confident nurse to speak up and challenge a time-pressed surgeon. After all, the surgeon is probably very experienced and the correct patient and procedure were probably already confirmed in the pre-op area by another nurse—unless he was also pressed for time.

Pre-operative sponge counts by two nurses (or a nurse and a surgical tech) are required to ensure a correct baseline count before surgery begins. During surgery, each sponge brought into the operative field is logged on a board and a tally of used sponges is reconciled at the end of the procedure before closing the patient. Of course, the entire process breaks down if the initial count was inaccurate. The first experienced nurse had been through the drill hundreds of times without an error so there was probably minimal risk when the second required person slipped off to perform some other necessary pre-surgical task. No one has ever miscounted, right?

Administration of potentially dangerous medication requires the presence of two healthcare providers for a read-back to confirm the correct patient is receiving the prescribed medication in the proper dose. Occasionally busy providers trusting each other to do the job properly dispense with the read-back. What could possibly go wrong if a newborn infant in the neonatal ICU receives an adult concentration or another baby's potent medication?

As a Risk Manager who investigated multiple examples of each of these scenarios, the common thread was a skilled team member trusted a known experienced colleague to do the job correctly. Usually because the team member felt time pressure to do other tasks. In the rush of the moment, the communication protocol was rationalized as unnecessary and "probably safe this time." What the field of risk assessment and mitigation reminds us is communication protocols exist for a reason. We are all human; all human beings make mistakes.

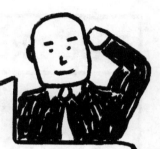

Do This

Follow all required communication protocols

Have the courage to speak up when needed

Consciously slow down, especially when busy

Remember we are all human and we will err

Don't Do This

Blindly trust familiar experienced colleagues

Gamble with patient safety even one time

Rationalize violating established protocols

Assume the other person has done their job

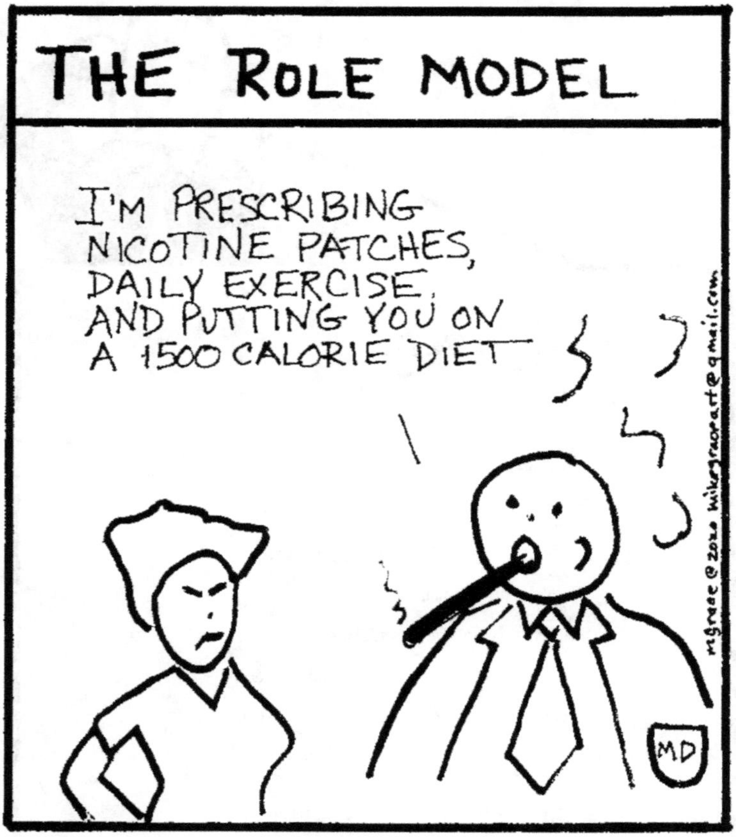
THE ROLE MODEL
I'M PRESCRIBING NICOTINE PATCHES, DAILY EXERCISE, AND PUTTING YOU ON A 1500 CALORIE DIET
MD
mgrace ©2020 mikegraceart@gmail.com

14

The Testimonial

IN THIS CHAPTER

Patients' investigation of their healthcare providers should prompt providers' self-evaluation and improvement when needed.

Nurses and doctors learn credibility, trustworthiness, and likeability are key attributes sought by patients.

When advertising agencies launch a new ad campaign, one of their popular strategies is the testimonial. As consumers we see testimonials all the time in both print and electronic media. The spokesperson may be a familiar celebrity or an unknown personality but they all possess a certain credibility of character. Whether it's anti-wrinkle cream from a pretty model or a reverse mortgage from an aging actor, they all command our attention. They convey a sense of trustworthiness, authority, and likability. Their presence is persuasive and we often succumb to their Message. These are the Ultimate Senders.

Healthcare providers need to become Ultimate Senders of the Messages they relate to their Receivers. They need to be credible, trustworthy, and likable. That is—if they want to positively impact their patient audience. And in my experience, no one enters the healing arts without a desire to help others and make a positive impact on their chosen profession.

Like it or not, the pressure to meet the consuming public's high expectations has never been greater—fueled by internet research and slick media. Patients routinely consult physician and hospital consumer websites to make decisions who to see and where to go. Their satisfaction with a recent hospitalization is measured by post-discharge governmental surveys. Healthcare delivery systems look at physician and nurse performance. Insurance companies track patient experience. We're awash in data and social media opinions. All providers are being evaluated by others. It is incumbent on the provider to do a bit of self-analysis. How do I really come across? Do patients find me credible, trustworthy, and likable? In other words, would I be hired for a testimonial?

- Credibility springs from inner confidence. You know what you're talking about. You speak confidently with quiet assurance. This is not the same as boasting. Confidence comes from knowledge, experience and education. Admitting you're not perfect can be a virtue. Few things are as attractive as humility. Admitting you are still learning inspires confidence, especially in the dynamic, ever-changing world of medicine. Credibility also comes from modeling the behaviors you espouse. No one believes a hypocrite. And as the saying goes: "No one buys a diet from a fat man."
- Trustworthiness comes from truth-telling. Don't promise what you can't deliver. Candidly acknowledge no one can guarantee a specific medical outcome. Be up front about risks and benefits. Be clear and consistent in the Messages you deliver. Always follow-through on what you promise.
- Baby-faced new doctors have special challenges to establish trustworthiness. Don't dissemble about your lack of experience. Poke fun at your youthful appearance. Honesty is disarming and refreshing. But as a newly minted doctor, your knowledge about the most current medical science is probably greater than many more experienced practitioners. And older doctors, perhaps those nearing retirement, shouldn't shy away from mentioning their on-going education to stay current with medical knowledge and the latest surgical techniques.
- Likeability is simply being a nice person—warm, kind, caring, friendly, and interested in others. Patients actually expect their providers—doctors and nurses—to be human, approachable, and empathetic. In fact, 65% of patient satisfaction has been attributed to physician empathy.[24] The "old school" notion of the emotionally remote doctor dispensing advice to the appropriately appreciative patient may never have been true, but it certainly is not the current state of medical practice.

---

[24] Stone, J., "The Importance of Empathy in Healthcare: Advancing Humanism," Medical GPS, 2019

Admittedly, those physicians in non-patient centered fields like pathology don't face quite the same expectations of likability, at least from patients. But it's probably a trait much appreciated by their peers and work colleagues! However, for doctors with regular patient contact, such as pediatricians, it should come as no surprise the number one trait sought in a new pediatrician is "warm and friendly."[25]

Before the public's obsession with ratings, it was the presumed and tolerated stereotype that surgeons lacked proper bedside manners. "If they were good with a knife, they were good enough." No longer. Surgical specialties—general, orthopedic, cardiac, neurosurgical—have the highest volume of insurance malpractice claims among all medical groups according to a national benchmarking report released in 2019.[26] It seems the public is looking for more than operating room skills. Pre- and post-operative contact with a likable and approachable surgeon is also important.

Regardless of specialty and medical outcome, claims data reveals this truth—it is easier for a patient to sue a doctor they don't really know than one they have come to hold in high personal regard. It makes sense. From the outset, did the doctor forge a team spirit with the patient and family? Did everyone have a sense they were pulling together to attain the same goal? Did the doctor take the time to share his humanity? If so, the patient will think twice before suing. On the other hand, who cares about someone no more tangible than the blur of a white coat racing between examination rooms?

---

[25] Levinson, W., "Doctor-patient communication and medical malpractice: implications for pediatricians," Pediatric Annals, 1997 Feb 28; 26(3): 186–193

[26] CRICO Strategies, "Malpractice risk in communication failures," 2015 Annual Benchmarking Report, Boston, MA: The Risk Management Foundation of the Harvard Medical Institutions, Inc., 2015

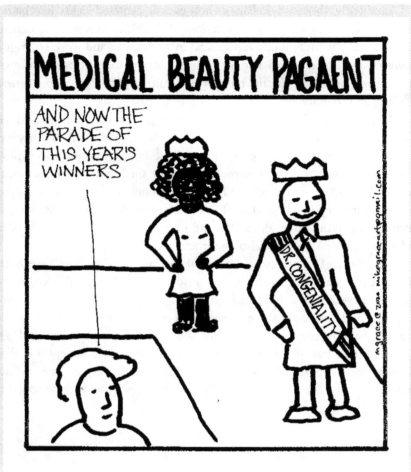

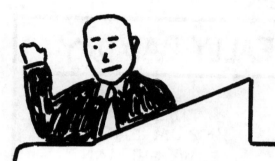

MEDICAL BEAUTY PAGAENT
AND NOW THE PARADE OF THIS YEAR'S WINNERS
DR. CONGENIALITY
mikegraceart@gmail.com

Do This

Engage in self-analysis how you come across

Project credibility with confidence

Model the behaviors you espouse

Project trustworthiness by always being truthful

Show your humanity by affable friendliness

Don't Do This

Boast about your accomplishments

Guarantee a specific medical outcome

Mislead about your lack of experience

Remain emotionally detached

Fail to get to know your patients

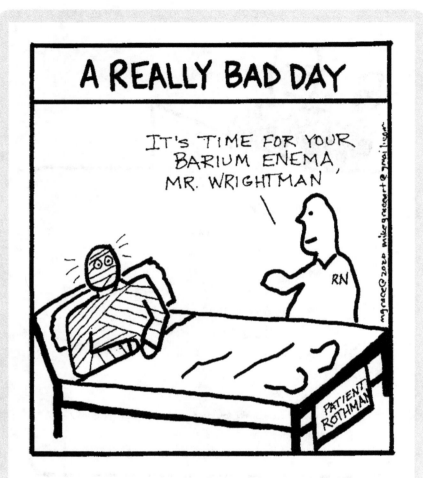

15

Patient Preparation for the Office Visit

IN THIS CHAPTER

Patients are given recommendations of best practices for a productive office visit.

Nurses and doctors should encourage patients to keep current medication lists, and to come to the encounter with an agenda of their concerns and notes about their medical condition.

As we've seen, communication is never one-sided. In healthcare, while great responsibility for effective dialogue falls on the doctor and nurse, patients have much to do themselves to enhance the communication encounter.

Always know what type of provider encounter you're getting into. Are you scheduling a visit for a focused physical complaint or an annual wellness check? Different amounts of time are scheduled by the doctor's office staff depending on the purpose of the visit. Don't be afraid to ask the receptionist how much time will be allotted with the doctor. Once your expectations are in alignment with reality, you can better prepare. And you won't be so surprised or as irritated if you're politely told to refocus on the purpose of the visit.

No matter the length of the scheduled office visit, here is your to-do list:[27]

- Come prepared with a list of current medications. Cell phone camera photos of each pill container label are a quick and efficient way to capture this information. This is much easier than writing out the properly spelled name

---

[27] US Dept of Health & Human Services, National Institute on Aging, "How to Prepare for a Doctor's Appointment," www.nia.nih.gov/health/how-prepare-doctors-appointment

of each drug, dosage, use, and prescriber. You should know the purpose of each medication and approximately how long you have been taking it. Don't forget to include non-prescribed vitamins and herbals you take on a regular basis. In certain dosages, these can potentially have an adverse effect on health and interact with prescribed medications.

- Make notes about the onset and development of your condition by date and time. Healthcare providers are always focused on timelines and the degrees of severity of all symptoms.
- Know your family history, especially as it may relate to your current complaints.
- Create an agenda and bring a written list of questions with you. The stress of the moment and the rush of the visit may cause you to forget everything you wanted to discuss. This advance preparation will help you to relax and focus.
- If you have done internet research about your suspected medical problem bring it with you. But be aware "armchair diagnoses" are often incorrect and the internet is full of inaccurate and inapplicable medical information.
- Arrive 15–20 minutes before your scheduled appointment. Typically, your doctor will have forms to update about health history, insurance coverage, and personal contact information. Arriving late for the appointment will likely cut into your face time with the provider.

Once in the encounter, listen carefully to the healthcare providers' questions and answer them directly and truthfully without getting off-topic. This includes questions from the entire medical team—the medical assistant, nurse, and doctor. Remember, the accuracy of the doctor's diagnosis and the efficacy of her treatment plan are only as good as the information on which they are based. Bringing a trusted friend or family member with you to the office visit can later serve as a useful sounding board about details of the meeting.

Finally, don't hesitate "to correct the record" if the provider has misunderstood you and respectfully question anything you don't understand. It is never inappropriate to inquire about the doctor's prior experience with any recommended treatment or procedure, the pros and cons of any recommendation, the available alternatives, and the likelihood of success. You should never feel pressured to sign any documents or make instantaneous decisions. Listen to your inner voice. If it doesn't sound right or feel right, it probably isn't right for you. Never hesitate to get a second medical opinion.

Do This

Create a written agenda of questions/concerns

Keep a current list of all medications

Make a timeline of medical events and symptoms

Bring relevant internet research

Clarify any points of confusion

Don't Do This

Come unprepared for any medical encounter

Waste providers' time by getting off topic

Evade providers' questions

Fail to silence your cell phone during the visit

Fail to speak up about problems/concerns

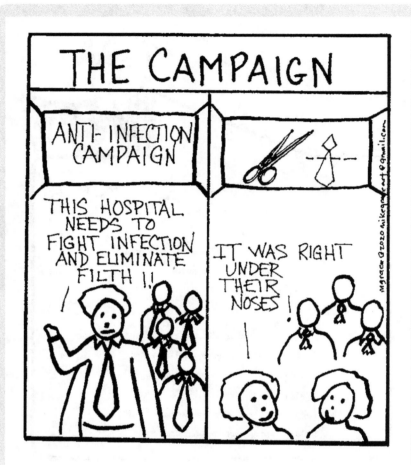

16

Patient Preparation for the Hospital Stay

IN THIS CHAPTER

Patients are provided guidance about hospital work flow and useful tips to improve communication during their hospital stay.

Nurses and doctors are reminded of pivotal moments when miscommunication is most likely such as shift handoffs, patient identification procedures, and the discharge process.

If you are going to the hospital, understanding the work flow will prevent confusion and frustration. During an Emergency Department visit, you will see a team of providers, starting with a triage nurse who will prioritize the severity of your case in comparison with other patients waiting to be seen. Eventually, you'll meet the emergency physician who is usually part of a group which has a contract with the hospital.

We have all been questioned by ED personnel. But we often fail to appreciate their triage decisions and medical diagnoses are largely based on patient history including onset, duration, and severity of symptoms. This information can also affect the scope of examination and the types of testing. ED providers love timelines and specific facts as much as primary care doctors. Get your facts straight and, whenever the situation allows, write them down. Hopefully you stored the pictures of all your medications on your cell phone because the ED will also require that information.

We all know there are barriers to effective communication including pain, fear, and confusion. Especially in the traumatic setting of an emergency department. If possible, come to the ED with a friend or family member who, with your permission, can be your advocate and surrogate spokesperson.

Returning to the ED within hours or days means you'll be restarting the communication process all over with a new cast of characters. Yes, the first ED group made notes in the computer but plan on verbally rehashing everything again from the beginning, including any interval changes since the last visit. This is when you are really going to appreciate having made those notes! If you are referred to the ED by your primary care physician, don't expect that person to meet you at the hospital or even necessarily speak with the ED team. The major responsibility for an accurate history is on your shoulders! Remember, inaccurate history can lead to incorrect diagnosis and ineffective treatment.

If you are admitted into the hospital, you will encounter a new set of doctors, probably a group of hospitalists who also have a contract with the hospital. They specialize in the care of admitted patients. However, don't expect to see the same doctor every day. On the contrary, typically you will seldom see the same doctor twice.

In theory, the first shift's off-going hospitalist gives report to the next shift's on-coming hospitalist about each patient's condition. And in theory, the new hospitalist consults the electronic medical record to get up to speed about what has already been done by other providers. Unfortunately, some electronic healthcare systems are fragmented and compartmentalized meaning one hospital group or department may lack access to records made by another group or department. And in most electronic medical record systems there is some time delay before all documents get into the system.

What does this rotating carousel of changing doctors and inaccessible records mean for your hospitalization? You are going to be constantly asked to repeat what's been done and how you're feeling.

- As with your doctor office visits, come to the hospital with written notes including a timeline of events and a list of medications.
- Always have a patient advocate. You will get better and more consistent care if the doctors and nurses know someone is looking out for you.
- It is advisable practice for you or your advocate to keep a journal of every encounter in the hospital. It will function as a living diary of events to be consulted throughout the hospital stay. The journal is the most efficient way to cut through patient-provider miscommunication. Make sure each journal

entry is timed and dated and contains the name and specialty of everyone you meet. Be careful about gender stereotyping. Not all doctors are men and not all nurses are women.

The continuity of your care will largely come through the nursing staff. Unlike the hospitalists who may make an appearance once a day, the nurses are your lifeline around the clock. And while the same nurse may not work multiple consecutive days, they will become known to you and be the most familiar with your care.

Like hospitalists, the off-going shift nurse should give report about your condition to the on-coming shift nurse. Best practice is for this to occur at your bedside and for you to participate in the communication process. If this is not being done, ask to participate! Hand-off communication errors are a major source of patient harm.[28] Don't hesitate to speak up if a nurse has misunderstood something about your condition. Smart doctors understand nurses are their eyes and ears; when they want to know what is really happening with their patient, they talk to the nurse.

While in the hospital, you will encounter all types of healthcare workers in addition to nurses and certified nurse's aides. These include phlebotomists, respiratory and physical therapists, dietitians, transporters and x-ray technicians, to name only a few. None of them know you. Therefore, all hospitals have devised a three-part system properly to identify patients by full name, date of birth, and medical record number. This is the same information printed on your wristband at the time of admission.

- No one in the hospital should give you any medication or treatment, or even take you out of your room, without first verifying your identity by all three patient identifiers. The only proper way to obtain this information from a conscious patient is by asking open-ended questions: For example: "What is your full name and date of birth?" And then the questioner should compare the ID number on the wristband with the ID number on the doctor's order. Asking leading questions, especially of a groggy patient who will often defer to the "authority figure," leads to inaccurate nods of assent. (For example: "You are Nicholas Romanov, date of birth 2-18-1972, correct?")

---

[28] The Joint Commission, "Inadequate hand-off communication," Sentinel Alert Event, Issue 58, 2017 Sept 12

- The three patient identifier system must ALWAYS be followed. The failure to comply is serious; the wrong patient receives treatment intended for someone else. Obviously, this is potentially life-threatening. All patients must actively participate in this aspect of their care and hold all healthcare workers accountable for strict adherence to this essential hospital regulation.
- Literally every month in the hospital I investigated multiple examples of lapses in the three patient identifier system. Wrong patients were taken from their rooms by careless transporters and blood was drawn on the wrong person by rushing phlebotomists. Keep in mind, at any given time hospitals have multiple patients with the same name—Johnsons and Rodriguezes abound. During one week we had 3 patients with the identical first, middle, and last names!

Finally, you will discover that long before you leave the hospital, there will be numerous conversations with case managers, nurses, doctors, social workers, and family members about the continuum of care at your next destination whether it is home, a rehabilitation location, or a skilled nursing facility. The Centers of Medicare and Medicaid Services has designed a system of financial "carrots and sticks" geared to grab the attention of the hospital with the goal you not be readmitted within 30 days of discharge. To that end, anticipate being questioned about your social support system and any barriers to recovery. Miscommunication among any of the participants is likely to land you back in the hospital thereby compromising your health and delaying recovery.

Discharge misunderstandings are rampant. A University of Kansas study revealed patient understanding of medication side effects at the time of discharge was substantially less than what their doctors perceived. Doctors thought 89% of their patients understood whereas only 57% of patients said they understood. [29] What to do? Doctors need to use feedback loops to verify accurate understanding. Patients need to speak up about any confusions no matter how rushed they feel to leave the hospital.

Who do you talk to if things go wrong or if your needs are not being met at any stage of your hospitalization? Always start with the person involved. We've learned there can be many explanations why things go awry. Of course,

---

[29] Agency for Healthcare Research and Quality (AHRQ), "Strategy 6G: Training to Advance Physicians' Communication Skills," 2017 July, https.//www.ahrq.gov/sites/default/files/wysiwyg/cahps/quality-improvement/improvement-guide/6-strategies-for-improvement

such communication should be private and respectful mirroring the best practices we've outlined.

But if that doesn't work, you have a few options. If the issue involves a nurse, go up the nursing chain of command—shift supervisor, charge nurse, or floor nursing director. Some of them may already have come by your room to introduce themselves. At night, ask for the Nursing House Supervisor. If it's a hospitalist or emergency physician issue, again follow the chain of command by asking to speak with the head of the hospitalist or ED group or, alternatively, the hospital's Chief Medical Officer.

Apart from these resources, you are always at liberty to speak with the institution's Patient Relations Officer or Ombudsman. Still have a problem? Call the hospital's Risk Manager or Patient Safety Officer.

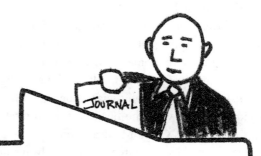

Do This

Keep a daily hospital journal

Always have a family member/friend advocate

Participate in nursing change of shift handoffs

Immediately clarify misunderstandings

Actively engage in the discharge process

Don't Do This

Let the hospital ignore proper ID procedures

Assume healthcare providers are always right

Assume the medical record is current or accurate

Assume others will make your history/needs known

Fail to speak up about problems/concerns

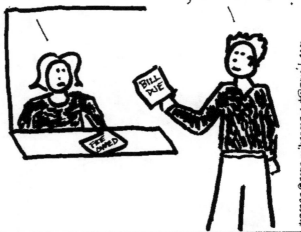

17

The Angry Patient

IN THIS CHAPTER

Patients identify with frustration during doctor office visits and appreciate achievable solutions.

Nurses and other allied healthcare professionals recognize the importance of taking an efficient history, reading non-verbal cues, and diffusing patient dissatisfaction.

Doctors are reminded they are responsible for the conduct of their office staff and how to respond to an angry patient.

Let's explore a common situation in the doctor's office which is guaranteed to raise the blood pressure of most patients.

For the third day in a row, Mrs. O'Donnell wakes up feeling miserable. Feverish, headachy, with an upset stomach. She thinks to herself: "I've got to see the doctor. I'm not getting better." She calls the office of her primary care physician, a female internist she's been treating with for several years. "Hello, Mrs. O'Donnell here. I desperately need to see Dr. Mohammed today if possible. I think I have the flu. I feel rotten and I think I'm getting worse." The schedule is full but the receptionist says: "No problem. How about 3:15? Please show up 15 minutes early so we can have you fill out paperwork."

Mrs. O'Donnell arrives promptly at 3pm. The waiting room is full. She reads and completes the medical history form. "Purpose of visit—flu?" "Symptoms—fever, headache, upset stomach." "On a 10 point scale, rate the severity of each symptom." She complies. "Duration—3 days." "Treatments—aspirin and the pink stuff for my stomach." She hands in the form.

3:15 comes and goes. 3:30. 3:45. 4:00. At 4:10, Mrs. O'Donnell is finally called back to an exam room and greeted by the smiling medical assistant. "And why are you here to see us today?" "I think I have the flu," she tersely replies. "And how long have you believed this to be the case?" "About 3 days, maybe 4. I don't remember." "And what are your symptoms and please rate them for me on a scale of 1 to 10 with 10 being the worst." At this point, Mrs. O'Donnell explodes: "Dearie, don't you read that damn form? I've waited over an hour to get in here and I'm feeling worse by the minute." Again, the medical assistant smiles: "I have just a few more questions and then the doctor will see you. And what treatments have you taken?"

At 4:30, Dr. Mohammed enters the room. "What a pleasure to see you again, Mrs. O'Donnell. It's only been, what a month, since I last saw you. What brings you in today?" Predictably, the patient unloads and regales the unsuspecting physician with a litany of her perceived mistreatment.

As we will see, there were a number of missed opportunities for more effective communication:

- The receptionist should have made clear to Mrs. O'Donnell there were no available appointments that day. Much better to be truthful and set realistic expectations from the outset. "Dr. Mohammed is fully booked today. However, I know you are one of her long-time patients. We could try to fit you in between other patients but you'll probably have to wait. Would that be acceptable or shall we try for tomorrow?"
- The front desk should offer any patient who has waited longer than 15–20 minutes for the scheduled visit the option of rescheduling. Everyone wants to feel they have some measure of control. "I'm sorry. But as you can see, the doctor is running unavoidably behind. We know your time is valuable. May we reschedule or do you prefer to continue waiting?
- The medical assistant should have begun the encounter with an apology. "I'm sorry we've kept you waiting so long." And she should have acknowledged the patient's ill health with an expression of compassionate sympathy.
- The medical assistant should have acknowledged having received and reviewed the medical history form before asking any questions. "I have your form in front of me. I see you are here for the flu. Are there any other chief medical concerns today?" Questions should be clarifying, not repetitive.

"Have you thought of anything else to add to your answers on the form? If not, I'll enter the information in the record." Asking identical questions is seldom productive and always irritating, especially to people who are not feeling well. Have a reason for asking about the answers. For example, "Do you recall the brand name of the stomach medication? Perhaps it was Pepto-Bismol or Maalox?" Restatement of the same questions and the same answers is a time-waster.

- The medical assistant was untrained in reading verbal and non-verbal body language. She should have acknowledged rather than ignored the patient's frustration before it reached a boiling point. Everyone wants to feel heard and understood.

- The medical assistant should have alerted the doctor an angry patient was waiting for her. There is never a reason for staff to allow the provider to walk blindly into a minefield.

- The doctor should have entered the room with a sincere apology on her lips. Patients' time is no less valuable than doctors' time.

- The doctor should always be aware of the reason for the patient's visit before the encounter. There is a reason for collecting information from the patient in the history questionnaire and from the medical assistant. Time savvy physicians will use those resources and not reinvent the proverbial wheel by a rehash of identical information from the patient.

- Once the patient is hopping mad, there is no point in arguing or mounting a defense.[30] Listen. Acknowledge. Apologize.

---

[30] Huntington, B., "Communication Gaffes: a root cause of malpractice claims," Proceedings, (Baylor Univ Medical Center), 2003 April; 16(2): 157, 159

Do This

Give the patient realistic time expectations

Offer the long-waiting patient time to reschedule

Train staff to coordinate information gathering

Train staff to respond to verbal and non-verbal cues

Listen to complaints, acknowledge, and apologize

Don't Do This

Waste patients' time

Engage in redundant information gathering

Ignore warning signs the patient is angry

Fail to acknowledge the patient's feelings

Fail to warn the doctor the patient is upset

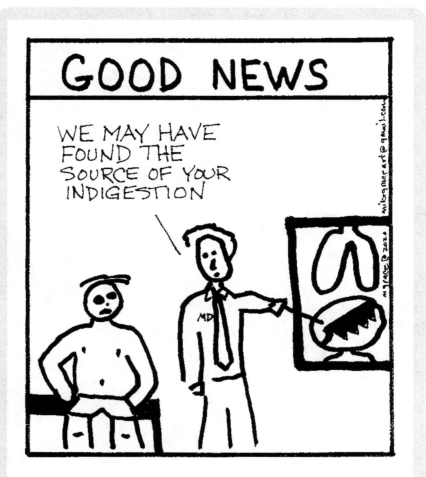

18

The Quiet Patient

IN THIS CHAPTER

Patients, nurses and doctors learn about identifiable persons who are prone to be quiet during medical encounters and suggested strategies to help them open up.

Make any patient angry enough and he'll find his voice. But some patients by nature are more reticent than others. These taciturn patients require some special effort to obtain a thorough history.

Who are we talking about? Anyone who appears to be holding back. These are people who respond with terse, evasive, and monosyllabic answers. While any patient could certainly fall into this situation, research has thrown some light on demographic categories of the frequently taciturn patient.[31,32] At the risk of grossly stereotyping and offending the exceptions, here they are:

- Men of any age. We don't go to the doctor as often as women. And when we see a doctor it is often only at the prodding of a spouse or family member.
- Young people under the age of 18. They have not personally selected the provider so they feel no personal allegiance or rapport. And generational

---

[31] National Center for Health Statistics, *Summary Health Statistics Tables for U.S. Adults: National Health Interview Survey, 2018*, Table A-18c

[32] National Center for Health Statistics, *Summary Health Statistics Tables for U.S. Children: national Health Interview Survey, 2018*, Table C-8c

differences of language and perception of "old people" inhibit frank discussion, especially of a sensitive nature.

- Members of minority groups, racial or ethnic. Too often, especially for new encounters, there is a reticence to speak candidly to a distrusted "authority" figure.

Once such patients are identified, what tools are available to the doctor or nurse provider?

- This is the time for open-ended questions which call for a narrative response. These include the classic journalist questions Who? What? When? Where? Why? How? And their variations: "What do you mean by that?" "What else do you remember?"
- Then politely ask for more information. "Please explain." "Tell me more." "I'd like to hear about that."
- Listen to the narrative response without interrupting. Even if the patient is getting off topic. Once the taciturn patient is talking, the direction of the patient's statements may give you some insight into her behavior and the meaning behind the words.
- Acknowledge what you're hearing. For example, a teenager may mumble: "It's personal. You wouldn't understand." You might reply: "It's my job to hear about personal things. Everything you say is just between us. I talk with teenagers all the time. Why don't you give me a try?"
- Acknowledge your impression that the patient is holding back information. "Am I correct you're not telling me something important?" "Why don't you want to talk about it?" Here is where "reading" the silence is key. As the saying goes: "People who don't understand your silence will never understand your words."
- With the patient's permission, try to get a family member in the room with both of you. "Is your wife here with you today? Do you mind if we ask her to join us?" Having either the person who prompted the visit or a knowledgeable or trusted person in the room as part of the history taking can add valuable information. And hopefully put the patient at greater ease.
- As a last-ditch effort, you can always try to bluff! This is a tactic used by trial lawyers who pretend to know something when we have no proof. For example, confidently ask: "Tell me about your health worries." Rather than,

"Do you have any health concerns?" which is likely to produce a simple negative response. The confident question assuming the truth of the fact is designed to mislead the person into believing you already know the answer so further denial is pointless.

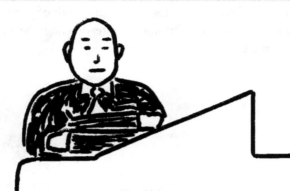

Do This

Recognize the patient who is holding back

Read the patient's silence

Tactfully confront the patient's behavior

Use open-ended questions to gain information

Encourage knowledgeable family to participate

Don't Do This

Ignore demographic groups of such patients

Ignore the patient's silence

Ask "yes" or "no" questions

Interrupt once the patient is talking

Fail to bluff when all else fails

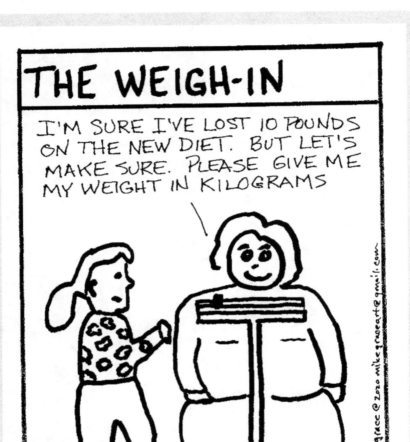

19
The Unfocused Patient

IN THIS CHAPTER

Patients, nurses and doctors learn about unfocused persons who tend to be distracted during medical encounters and suggested strategies to help them concentrate on the matter at hand.

The unfocused, distracted, and chatty patient presents a special set of challenges. If unchecked, the patient, not the provider, ends up controlling the encounter but seldom achieves the purpose of the visit. If it is an established patient, the provider has the benefit of a "heads-up" of what's likely to occur. If it is a new encounter, the provider is going to need to be nimble on his feet. Here are some effective strategies:

- Set the patient's time expectations from the outset. Train the office staff to educate patients about the length of the scheduled visit—usually 15 minutes for a focused visit and 50 minutes for an annual wellness check.
- Read your patient's body language and affect from the outset. The unfocused, distracted and chatty person often arrives excitedly bouncing from one unrelated topic to the next. It could be the morning traffic, a headline in the newspaper, or a grandchild's upcoming graduation. Give them a couple of minutes to wax poetic on whatever topic they want. And bite your tongue and don't interrupt. Such persons often need to let off some steam before they can settle down.

- After the exchange of greetings and the expiration of their "free time," briefly acknowledge what you've heard. "Yes, I can see why you're so proud of your granddaughter." Then get down to business by reminding the patient of the purpose of the visit. "I understand you've been experiencing some insomnia lately. Let's talk about that."

- Keep your questions focused and brief. Start with the narrative questions. Then quickly become more pointed with questions calling for "yes" or "no" answers. Proceed as necessary to any needed examination and testing and then move on to the diagnosis and recommended treatment plan.

- Answer the patient's questions, but keep your responses concise. The longer you talk, the more likely the patient will get distracted. Such persons are often positively influenced by pictures and diagrams in patient brochures. Show them the pictures or diagrams to reinforce your message rather than repeating what you've said.

- When you sense the patient is becoming distracted, say her name. Research indicates we all significantly refocus attention when we hear our names spoken out loud. But don't overdo it. Beginning each sentence with the patient's name will make them immune to the strategy.[33]

- When the unfocused patient wanders off topic, acknowledge what they've said but reel them back in. "Well, I'm sorry to hear that in addition to the insomnia, you also think you have some sleep apnea. But we would need more time than we have today to address that problem. I'd be happy for you to come back to see me about it in the near future. But today let's stay focused on the insomnia."

- With the unfocused patient, it is particularly important for the provider to use a feedback loop to confirm the patient has heard and understood the treatment plan and any verbal instructions they've been given. "So, Mr. Horowitz, when you fill the prescription I just gave you, tell me how many pills you are going to take and when."

- With any patient, but particularly the unfocused ones, get a verbal promise they will do what you have asked. Not just a nod of the head but actual articulation. "Promise me you'll fill the prescription today." "Yes, I will." Research shows we are more likely to follow through on a commitment if it is said out loud. Our brains hear what our mouths say.[34]

---

[33] Schulz, J., "Using a person's name in conversation," Michigan State University Extension, 2017 Jan 12

[34] Tesema, M., "4 Science-Backed Reasons to Say Your Self—Talk Out Loud," Shine, 2020 Sept 18, https://www.advice.theshineapp.com/articles/4/science-backed-reasons-to-take-your-self-talk-out-loud/

This is a technique often used by trial lawyers when questioning prospective jurors. "This is obviously an emotional and tragic case involving the death of a young mother. But do you promise me you'll set aside any natural feelings of sympathy and follow His Honor's instructions and judge this case solely on the facts?" "Yes, I will."

- Reinforce the message by personally handing the patient written discharge instructions. Don't delegate this duty to your office staff. Review the instructions with the patient and answer any final questions. Confirm with a feedback loop what the patient should do if the condition worsens.

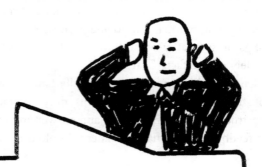

<u>Do This</u>

Communicate realistic time limitations

Give the patient a couple of minutes to unwind

Keep your questions and exam narrowly focused

Say the patient's name to get him refocused

Have the patient verbalize all agreements

<u>Don't Do This</u>

Allow the patient to control the encounter

Ask many open-ended questions

Give the patient long rambling explanations

Allow the patient to get off topic

Delegate the discharge process to another

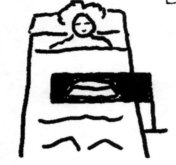
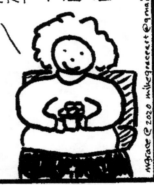

20
The Patient's Family

IN THIS CHAPTER

Patients learn about potential problems having family members involved in their medical care.

Nurses and doctors learn how to identify family members with whom they may share confidential patient information, how to interact with difficult family members, and which members are likely to be drivers of future litigation.

Frequently the patient's family is involved in the provider-patient encounter. As we've seen, this can be a benefit when a family member serves as the patient's advocate during hospitalization. And family members may also provide helpful information about a taciturn patient's history. But like most positives, there can be a negative flip side. Family members can be intrusive and disruptive to the doctor-patient relationship. As a consequence, many providers, especially doctors, mistakenly view family members as an irritant—persons who can be rightfully ignored. Nothing could be further from the truth. The patient may want them involved. But even the "uninvolved" may become future drivers of litigation on the patient's behalf.

At the outset, the doctor needs to verify whether she can legally speak with the family about the patient's confidential personal health information. The doctor must take her cue solely from the patient. "Who, if anyone, do you want to know your personal health information?" Then the doctor needs to document the chart accordingly.

Don't presume a wife wants her husband to know everything. Nor should adult children necessarily have access. Frequently families are fragmented with some adult children on the "outs" with the parents or each other. Understanding the "lay of the family land" is crucial, especially for the primary care provider. And don't presume an identified "contact person in the event of emergency" is intended to have access to personal health information.

It is a mistake to assume whoever followed the patient into the exam room is authorized to be there. The patient may have thought it too awkward to ask the person to remain in the waiting area. And just because someone is sitting at the hospital bedside does not necessarily mean the patient is comfortable with personal medical information being discussed. It has happened that a careless doctor wrongfully assumed a patient's spiritual counselor was a family member who would administer the prescribed suppository!

It is up to the doctor to figure out who's who and who has a right to be present. A good starting point is to inquire about the person's relationship with the patient. Is it a church elder? An adult only child? Or a visiting distant cousin? "Mr. Kim, may I speak freely in front of your son? Or would you prefer we talk confidentially one-on-one?"

What if the patient does not want a pushy family member to have access to personal health information? Here's a suggested strategy to avoid alienating the relative: "It was a pleasure meeting you, Mrs. Strong. However, I'm afraid my hands are tied. As much as I'd like to answer your questions, the law of patient confidentiality forbids me from doing so. If you were my patient, I'd be doing the same to protect your privacy. I'm sure you understand."

Once you know with whom you can legally speak, the potential complications of the family communication process are just beginning. Some patients' relatives just can't keep from interjecting themselves into the process. Even talkative patients can find themselves cut off by an adult child who supplies the answers. And some married people can't refrain from contradicting their spouses. Keep returning to your patient for the answers.

The goal, of course, is to get the patient's history from the patient (assuming mental competence) and then supplement the information from others whose insight may be pertinent. Here, some polite inquiry to the family member maybe warranted. "How often do you see or speak with the patient?" "Are you involved with her care?" "Do you attend other doctor visits?" The family member's responses can assist in determining the weight the doctor should give any proffered opinions. Make sure to document the history and attribute the source of information, especially anything contradictory.

A seldom appreciated fact is many lawsuits are instigated by family members.[35] Therefore, it is very important for the doctor to be polite to all, but especially to attend to the concerns of the involved family. For example, you may think you have already addressed all of the patient's questions about a recommended treatment, but the family's involvement means you may need to repeat what has already been said about risks, benefits, and alternatives. All family members' questions must be answered. If a family member advocates an alternative treatment, any surgical mishap or bad outcome will be blamed on the doctor. Under such circumstances, always encourage a second opinion. Just as you would do with a reluctant patient questioning your advice.

If the patient's health is failing, physician discussions with the approved family members become especially important. Don't assume they understand the prognosis and limited treatment options. This is the time to get everyone's expectations in alignment with medical reality. And document the discussion.

Here are a few predictors of litigation prone relatives:

- Did the patient die? If so, a future wrongful death suit must necessarily be brought by surviving heirs.
- Was the patient a child or grandchild of the family members? High emotions understandably run through such relationships.
- Did the patient or family have false expectations about the medical course? Groundless hopes for unrealistic outcomes fuel litigation.
- Was the patient permanently impaired, mentally or physically, by the medical treatment? Family members are more apt to become future litigation decision makers if the patient was seriously injured. However, perhaps surprisingly, a 2012 study found that poor people are less likely to sue than wealthier patients, probably due to a lack of legal resources.[36]
- Are the family members active caregivers of the patient? If so, they may have a financial reason to litigate.
- Did the patient or family members criticize another doctor? Persons with such overtly expressed opinions about prior medical care are more prone to sue.
- Are the family members millennials? People who reached adulthood in the early 21st century have a high expectation for healthcare and believe when it fails, someone should pay.[37]

[35] Hickson, O., Chayton, E., Githens, P., Sloan, F., "Factors that prompted families to file medical malpractice claims following perinatal injuries," JAMA, 1992; 267: 1359–1363

[36] McClellan, F., "Do Poor People Sue Doctors More Frequently? Confronting Unconscious Bias and the Role of Cultural Competency," Clinical Orthopaedics and Related Research, 2012 May

[37] Siegel, D., "Harnessing the power of medical malpractice data to improve patient care," ASHRM Journal of Healthcare Risk Management, 2019 Nov, 39(3): 36

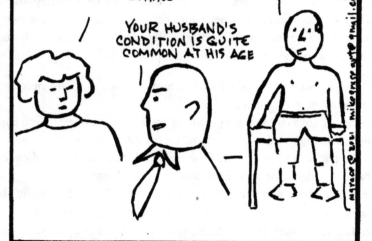

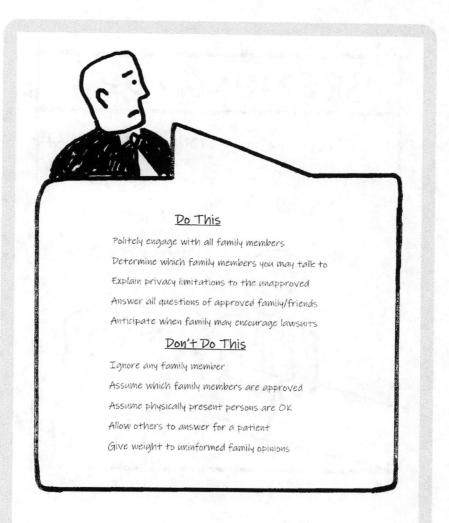

Do This

Politely engage with all family members

Determine which family members you may talk to

Explain privacy limitations to the unapproved

Answer all questions of approved family/friends

Anticipate when family may encourage lawsuits

Don't Do This

Ignore any family member

Assume which family members are approved

Assume physically present persons are OK

Allow others to answer for a patient

Give weight to uninformed family opinions

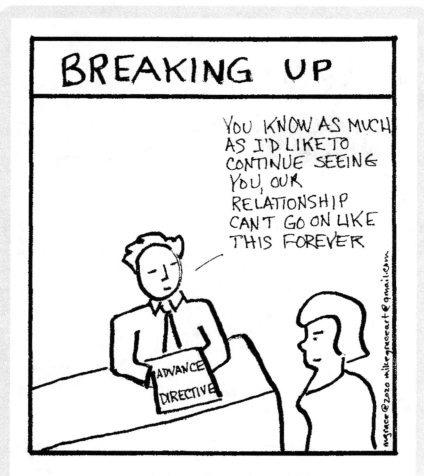

21
Legal Healthcare Documents

IN THIS CHAPTER

Patients learn about the two major types of healthcare documents and how to talk to their family members about end-of-life care.

Nurses and doctors learn which healthcare documents are pertinent and what situations trigger the role of a surrogate decision-maker.

There are some legal documents which define a physician's authority to act for a patient on the say-so of another person. Two of the most important are Durable Powers of Attorney and Advance Healthcare Directives.

A Durable Power of Attorney is a legal document giving authority over one's affairs to a third person. Powers of Attorney can be limited by subject matter—for example, to finances or to medical decisions. For our purposes, we are only concerned with Durable Powers of Attorney for Healthcare.

By their nature, such Powers of Attorney are *immediately effective* unless stated otherwise. They are always revocable at any time by the person conveying the authority to act. Each state has its own laws governing the exact content and form of the document. Most are notarized and witnessed by other parties whose signatures are affixed. Typically, the person accepting such a Power also signs agreeing to undertake the responsibility. The scope of the conveyed authority over healthcare decisions is specified in the document. For instance, there could be broad unlimited power over any healthcare decision or limited power confined to specified situations.

Durable Power of Attorney forms are widely available on the internet. However, you should always have them reviewed for completeness by an attorney practicing in your state to ensure all current legal requirements are met. Primary care physicians in particular should maintain a copy of the executed Durable Power of Attorney for Healthcare in the patient's medical chart.

The most commonly used legal document to set forth a person's healthcare desires are called Advance Healthcare Directives.[38] By their nature and as the title implies, these documents become effective *in the future* if you should be unable to make your own healthcare decisions. With the passage of the Affordable Care Act (Obamacare) the use of Advance Directives has become widespread. The federal government encourages physicians to have end-of-life conversations with their patients to ensure the patient's true wishes will be followed.

Like Powers of Attorney, Advance Directives are revocable at any time. Like Powers of Attorney, a specific person (and often an alternate) are identified as the surrogate decision-maker and a detailed list of end-of-life instructions are enumerated. For instance, the use of resuscitation, feeding tubes, and comfort care are typically addressed. Again, your physician should have a copy of the Advance Directive. If you haven't already created such a document, the next time you are treated in a hospital you will be offered an Advance Directive form to complete. It is easy to obtain such a form at any time from your primary care physician or local hospital.

Because Advance Directives are commonly used and revocable, patients upon admission to a hospital may have forgotten they already have one. There is always the potential more than one such document will be in the hospital's records or your physician's office. The last dated Advance Directive is the one which will apply to your future care. You may at different points in time have designated different people as your surrogate decision-maker. Again, the last dated document will control. It is always recommended to give the surrogate a copy of the Advance Directive as soon as you have signed it. If the new document includes the same surrogate but the nature of your end-of-life wishes has changed, ask the surrogate to destroy the out-of-date document. And don't forget to give an updated copy to your primary care physician.

---

[38] American Bar Association, "Giving Someone a Power of Attorney for Your Healthcare (multi-state guide and form)," 2020 Aug 25, https.//www.americanbar.org/groups/law_aging/resources/health_care_decsion_making/power__atty_guide_and_form_2011

Occasionally a surrogate decision-maker tries to "jump the gun" and become involved at the time of a hospitalization when the patient is still able to make her own medical decisions. This is not allowed. Everyone, including the physician, should only take direction from the patient. The role of surrogate decision-maker kicks in *only* when the patient can no longer decide for herself.

Everyone should talk to their family about their end-of life preferences. Let them know your wishes. Put it in writing and give them copies. Talking alone is never enough. A widow telling her four adult children she doesn't want a feeding tube to keep her alive will be heard and remembered differently. As we've learned, Messages are not always heard by the Receiver as intended by the Sender.

The result of undocumented end-of-life conversations can be an emotionally charged fight at the deathbed. Absent written direction, it will be up to the healthcare providers and the hospital administration to discern the patient's intention. As Risk Manager I was called more than once to referee a family's disagreement about their loved one's end-of-life care. Unfortunately, deference may be given to the loudest, most adamant family member, not the one who most accurately recalls mom's wishes.

Conversations with family members about death and dying are seldom easy. And, at times, egos can be bruised and arguments occur. Here is one suggested scenario for how the widowed mom can talk to her four adult children:

- "I want to talk to you about an important decision I've made about my last days if I'm unable to speak for myself. I don't expect you all to agree with me but I do expect you to honor my wishes. I don't want to be kept alive by machines. Just keep me comfortable. When it's my time, I'll be ready to go. I've put all the details in writing in this Advance Directive. I have copies for each of you. As you can see, I had to pick one person to speak for me and I've chosen Robin. I love you all and it was a hard choice. But I thought Robin would be best because she's a nurse and understands such things. She also lives closer than the rest of you, and frankly I know she's tough enough to "pull the plug." Please give her your support when the time comes."

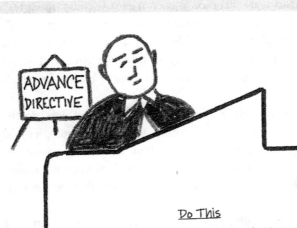

Do This

Have an Advance Directive for Healthcare

Give copies to your surrogate, doctor, and family

Discuss end-of-life decisions with your family

Don't Do This

Have more than one Directive

Let a surrogate decide if the patient can

Trust only verbal end-of-life decisions

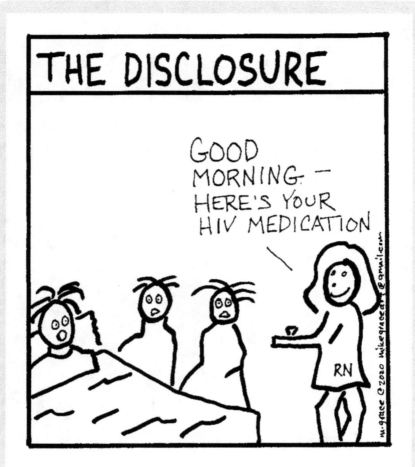

22
The Patient Bill of Rights

IN THIS CHAPTER

Patients, nurses and doctors learn about the 13 patient rights as well as potential consequences of ignoring them.

No healthcare provider—doctor or nurse—can speak appropriately to patients without understanding patient rights. Failure to respect patient rights can be grounds for a governmental investigation and possible hospital fines or discipline against the provider's medical or nursing license. Lack of adherence can also form the grounds for a patient lawsuit seeking monetary damages.[39]

Increasingly, patients and their family members are aware of these rights. For instance, any time a patient now enters the hospital, by federal regulation the admission paperwork must contain the Patient Bill of Rights. Note: there is no corresponding Doctor or Nurse Bill of Rights. This is patient centered care!

Here is a list of the 13 rights:

1. The right to appropriate medical care and humane treatment. Any medically necessary treatment must be given appropriate to the situation without discrimination, and human dignity must always be respected. In addition, medical emergencies must be treated irrespective of ability to pay.

---

[39] CMS Manual System Department of Health & Human Services (DHHS), Centers for Medicare & Medicaid. Services (CMS), Pub. 100-07 State Operations, Provider Certification, Transmittal 37, Date: 2008 October 17

2. The right to informed consent. A separate chapter is devoted to this important concept. Suffice it to say, all patients are entitled to be informed of the procedure, alternatives and risks with a right to refuse any medical treatment.

3. The right to privacy and confidentiality. While this topic is also the subject of a separate chapter, essentially a patient has the right to keep his personal health information confidential from anyone other than involved healthcare providers and insurers paying for treatment.

4. The right to information. The patient has the right to all test results and medical evaluations unless this information would be harmful to the patient such as a psychiatric report and then it must be released to an appropriate patient representative. The patient also has the right to review all itemized billing information.

   If the patient believes there are inaccuracies in his medical records or billing statements, federal statute and most state laws give the patient the right to request an amendment. Normally the request must be in writing specifying with particularity the record in question, the statements to be amended, and the reason for the request. The request must be granted unless the laws' provisions allow for a denial, such as the requested amendment would be factually in error. If the amendment is granted, the inaccurate information is generally not removed but the correction is added to the record.[40]

5. The right to choose a healthcare provider and facility. The patient has the right to hire his own doctor and to select a facility for treatment.

6. The right to self-determination. The patient has the right to decide what medical treatment will be received including end-of-life care.

7. The right to religious belief. An adult patient has the right to refuse treatment for religious reasons. Special circumstances may apply for minor children depending on the age and severity of illness.

8. The right to medical records. While the medical record belongs to the provider, the patient has a right to view and copy the record. Allowable costs and the timing of reproduction vary by state law.

9. The right to leave. A patient has the right to leave a facility at any time irrespective of medical condition so long as public health is not endangered.

---

[40] Privacy Act of 1974 (2020 edition), 5 USC, Section 552A, Individual's Right of Amendment (2–4) found online at www.justice.gov/opcl/privstat.htm

10. The right to refuse to participate in medical research. The patient has the right to be informed of any planned medical research and to refuse to participate.
11. The right to correspondence and to receive visitors. The patient has the right to receive mail and visitors subject to reasonable limits.
12. The right to express grievances. The patient has the right to complain about care without fear of reprisal and to be informed about the disposition of such complaint.
13. The right to be informed of his rights and obligations as a patient. The patient has the right to be informed of his legal rights and responsibilities.

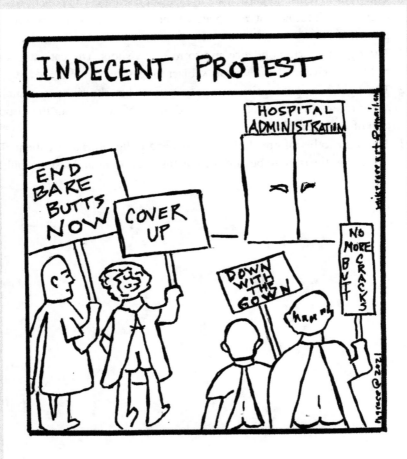

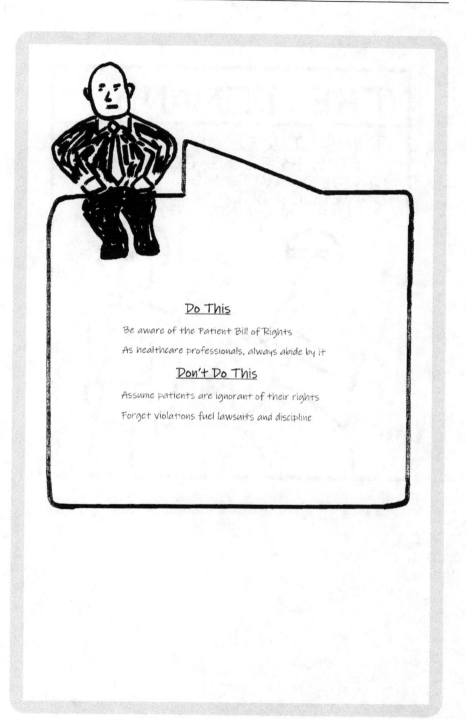

Do This

Be aware of the Patient Bill of Rights

As healthcare professionals, always abide by it

Don't Do This

Assume patients are ignorant of their rights

Forget violations fuel lawsuits and discipline

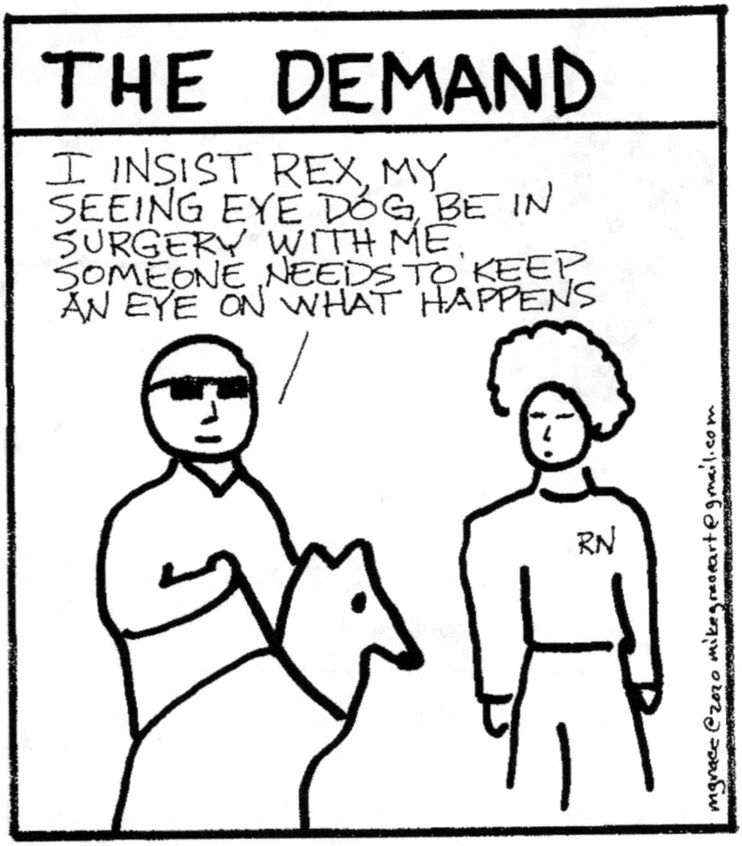
THE DEMAND
I INSIST REX, MY SEEING EYE DOG, BE IN SURGERY WITH ME. SOMEONE NEEDS TO KEEP AN EYE ON WHAT HAPPENS
RN
mgraec ©2020 mikegraecart@gmail.com

23

The Disabled Patient

IN THIS CHAPTER

Patients learn the Americans with Disabilities Act grants legal protections and affords legal remedies to ensure there is effective healthcare communication with the disabled population.

Nurses and doctors learn of recommended institutional procedures to implement the ADA as well as suggested strategies for communicating with blind, deaf and mute patients.

The Americans with Disabilities Act of 1990 fundamentally altered how society must treat persons with disabilities.[41] While the Act covers all types of physical and other disabling conditions, our focus is on those disabilities which impact communication—impairment of hearing, seeing, and speaking.

Interacting with patients who have communication disabilities should be treated like a legal emergency. From the very outset of the encounter, the healthcare provider will not be fulfilling the patient's legal rights if accommodation is not immediately made. Most of the rights enumerated within the Patient Bill of Rights require the ability to process information.

All hospitals and other large healthcare delivery systems have prepared for this situation. Typically, there are written institutional policies covering each step in the accommodation process—from computer solutions of video "face time" with sign language specialists to provision of written braille materials.

---

[41] Title III of the Americans with Disabilities ACT (1990), Section 504 of the Rehabilitation Act (1973)

Unfortunately, while not uncommon, healthcare workers don't deal with these situations often enough to have the details at their fingertips. This unfamiliarity can account for unacceptable delays and lead to avoidable lawsuits.

As a Risk Manager I was called upon to investigate numerous ADA problems. What follows is my personal list of ADA communication advice. As writer and wit Oscar Wilde noted: "The only thing to do with good advice is pass it on. It is never any use to oneself."

- Each institution needs a designated point person trained in ADA accommodation. This can be the Risk Manager, Patient Relations Officer, or member of the Administrative team. And there needs to be a designated "alternate" and identified "after hours" person.
- Everyone in the institution needs to be trained on the importance of prompt ADA accommodation, as well as the identity of the designated point persons and how to reach them.
- The point persons need to be told how to access the controlling written policies which are usually available in the institution's computer system. They also need to keep hard copies should the computer system shut down.
- The policies need to be highly specific including the "nuts and bolts" of implementing the accommodation strategy. For example, where are the "face time" computers or other materials kept? Who has the key to the room? What is the back-up plan if all machines are in use or are malfunctioning?
- Outside professional services exist for the provision of ADA accommodation to the mute, blind, and deaf population. Most institutions already have contracts with businesses which will provide electronic services. However, the institution also needs to vet the available in-person options in its geographic area. It should also pre-approve the point persons' authority to enter into a contract for on-site services if necessary. (For instance, if the hospital's own equipment is malfunctioning after hours.) There is no such thing as waiting to the next business day for CEO contract approval while a hospitalized deaf patient is in immediate need of cardiac surgery.
- The required accommodation is for all communication with all healthcare providers. It is not limited to only "significant" encounters as defined by the institution.
- The use of the patient's friends or family members without the patient's consent is not an acceptable substitute for professional services. It is imperative accurate communication of medical information, sometimes of a technical nature, is being appropriately conveyed.

- Keep in mind the ADA population is knowledgeable and sophisticated. They have been living with their disability and they know their rights, usually better than the healthcare providers. Often, they have an ADA advocate or attorney on "speed dial," needed resources as they have had to navigate through life. Violation of the Americans with Disabilities Act is a frequent source of litigation everywhere.
- Non-institutional healthcare providers like sole practitioners are not exempt from making reasonable accommodations for the disabled and need to plan accordingly. This may even involve going out-of-pocket to pay for a professional such as a sign language specialist. The ADA requires compliance from all practitioners who accept Medicare or Medicaid reimbursement.
- ADA patients often come to their medical encounters with "special needs" animals. Challenging their presence or demanding "proof" of the "special needs" status is inappropriate. Generally, the animal can accompany the patient, except in locations which pose an infection or other serious health risk. But accommodation does not mean medical staff has to take care of the animal. Walking and feeding are the sole responsibility of the patient.

Once the required ADA accommodation has been made for the person with a communication disability, there are a few basic strategies to keep in mind to maximize your effectiveness as a Sender of Messages.[42]

- For a person with a hearing or speaking loss, speak directly to the patient, not the sign language interpreter. Allow the interpreter time to translate before beginning your next thought. Speak without raising your voice or exaggerating your words. If the patient reads lips, keep your hand and objects away from your mouth and don't turn away or walk around while talking.
- For a person with a vision loss, introduce yourself and anyone with you. Use a normal tone of voice. Explain when you are leaving the environment. If the patient is accompanied by a service dog, don't pet or otherwise distract the animal unless the owner has given you permission.

---

[42] National League for Nursing, "Communicating with People with Disabilities," https.// www.nln.org/professional-development-programs/teaching-resources/ace-d/additional-resources/ communicating-with-people-with-disabilities#

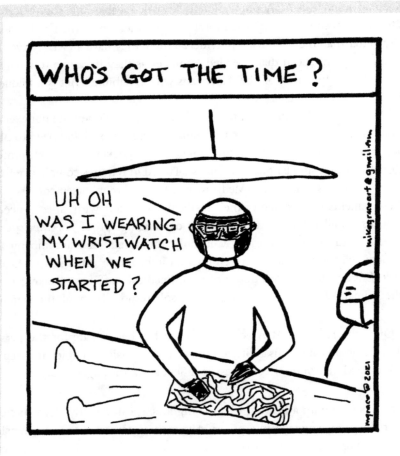

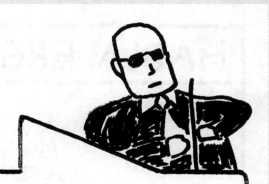

Do This

Become familiar with your duties under the ADA

Treat ADA communication as a legal emergency

Know your institution's accommodation protocols

Use professional 3rd parties unless waived

Don't Do This

Assume you are exempt from ADA rules

Fail to have a back-up plan for tech failures

Use minors or unapproved family to translate

Challenge the legitimacy of service animals

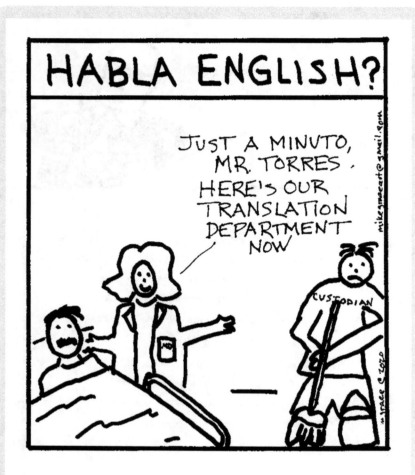

24
The Foreign Patient

IN THIS CHAPTER

Patients recognize the challenges of communicating when there are language and cultural differences.

Nurses are the focus of most institution's professional translation education and know to remind patients such services are free of charge.

Doctors learn the legal perils of ignoring professional translation services and are reminded of best communication practices with foreign language speakers from unfamiliar cultures.

In this chapter we are talking about differences in language or culture. Both present potential roadblocks to effective communication and opportunities for medical errors. As Sir William Osler, the "Father of Modern Medicine," reminded us: "It is much more important to know what sort of a patient has a disease than what sort of disease the patient has."

Non-English speaking patients can present many of the same challenges we've seen with disabled patients. Healthcare providers cannot properly proceed with care unless they can freely communicate with the patient. The Patient Bill of Rights demands nothing less. According to the 2010 U.S. Census, 20% of the population speaks a language other than English at home. Comic George Carlin mockingly appreciated our multi-lingual universe when he noted: 'Meow' means 'woof' in cat."

As with ADA policies, all hospitals and large healthcare organizations have anticipated caring for patients who speak dozens of foreign languages. Usually contracts have been entered into with electronic translation and interpretation services. Most include "face time" video options rather than the "old school" phone service. Just as we saw in treating "The Disabled Patient," there needs to be widespread education about the mechanics of the system including where equipment is stored and how it is accessed. And there needs to be a plan in place to deal with technical glitches. All non-English speaking patients need to be offered these services and reminded they are free of charge.[43]

Because language issues are so common, nursing is the logical place where most organizations have focused training. Education should include an emphasis on professional interpreters and use of the electronic translation system. It is never acceptable to rely on someone's half-forgotten high school French or German. While many nurses and nurse's aides speak fluent Spanish and Tagalog, relying on them for interpretation necessarily takes away from their nursing duties. But if existing staff is used, such person must be truly bilingual. There has to be a confidence medical concepts will not get garbled in translation. For the same reason, only adult family members and friends who are bilingual should be relied on. But, of course, only with the patient's consent. The foreign speaking patient may not want his nosey relative to know his confidential personal health information!

Physicians are probably the greatest barrier to the proper use of the institution's established translation policy. They are typically in a hurry and don't want to wait for a professional interpreter. They often find it easiest to pull in any available third party or proceed with a mixture of simple words and pantomime and hope for the best. But the doctor should beware—he is skating on thin legal ice. The more important the conversation, the greater the risk. If something goes wrong, the patient will claim, rightly or wrongly, she didn't understand. The best practice is for the physician to have the nurse trained in the institution's policy set up the electronic video call.

Once the electronic video connection is established, the physician should follow these best communication practices:

- Look at the patient, not the interpreter. Attention diverted away from the patient will miss non-verbal clues how the patient is feeling and what she means.

---

[43] The Joint Commission (TJC), *A Crosswalk of the National Standards for Culturally and Linguistically Appropriate Services (CLAS) in Health and Health Care*, 2014

- Use short sentences. Stop speaking after two or three sentences to give the interpreter the opportunity to translate. This takes practice to develop a rhythm where no one is interrupting the other speaker.
- If you are reading something to the patient, slow down. Most people read much faster than they speak. Inevitably the interpreter will fall behind and ask you to repeat what you've read.
- Don't hesitate to redirect the interpreter as necessary if you sense the patient is saying more than is being translated. "Please tell me every word the patient is saying."

Irrespective of language barriers, caring for a patient from an unfamiliar foreign culture is particularly tricky. In a polyglot society where people come from so many different places, it is a daunting task to become even superficially familiar with them all. Here are some effective approaches for dealing with the patient from a foreign culture:

- Always show respect for cultural differences, even those you don't understand. Everyone is proud of where they come from. And most people enjoy sharing their culture with others. Be patient and open to learning about their culture.
- Patients from different cultures may be unusually quiet. The caring physician needs to read the quietude. There is truth in the maxim: "Only those who care about you can hear you when you're quiet."
- When trying to get the quiet patient to open up, it is often helpful to begin with an "ice breaker" to establish rapport and common ground. For example, "Tell me a little bit about yourself." Knowing the patient just arrived in the country, or has been living in a refugee camp, or recently fled from a war zone, will give you better insight how to interact. Expressing an interest invites more expansive conversation. As the patient starts opening up, the suggestions in Chapter 18, "The Quiet Patient," may help.
- If the foreign patient is struggling to find the appropriate word in English, remain attentive. Don't interrupt and avoid the tendency to fill in the conversational gaps. When the patient is finished and if the provider is confused, use feedback immediately to clarify. "Did I understand correctly you've never previously been examined by a gynecologist?"
- Patients from different cultures, particularly some Asian or third world countries, may defer to authority and never overtly challenge or directly

disagree with the doctor. Silence does not mean agreement. Read the body language. And try to decipher the meaning behind a simple verbal response like "OK." Is the patient articulating real consent or simply responding in a manner he thinks the doctor wants to hear? Or is the patient's "OK" merely an acknowledgment of having heard the doctor's words without any intent to express agreement or disagreement?

- Some foreign patients may be culturally suspicious of authority figures, especially during an initial encounter. Again, read the verbal and non-verbal clues. You may find it useful to confront the issue directly. "I get the feeling you don't trust me. But I promise everything we say to each other is confidential. I cannot ethically share anything you tell me with the immigration authorities."

- Many women from conservative cultures may be uncomfortable speaking with a male provider much less be physically examined by one. Ask if she would prefer another female in the room, even during history taking.

- Encourage, with the patient's consent, the presence of first generation family members such as adult children who may assist in bridging the cultural divide. The "Americanized kids" can shed light on the parents' attitudes as well as their cultural norms, beliefs, and practices.

- If your community has a substantial population from a particular foreign country, take the time to learn a bit of the language and to educate yourself about the culture. The invested effort will pay dividends by improving doctor-patient-nurse communication. As South Africa's first post-apartheid president Nelson Mandela observed: "If you talk to a man in a language he understands, that goes to his head. If you talk to him in his language, that goes to his heart." Your interest and sensitivity may have the added benefit of building your medical practice within that ethnic community!

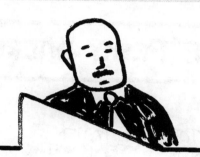

Do This

Use professional translation services

Be familiar with your institution's protocols

Speak slowly when using an interpreter

Show respect for cultural differences

Take the time to learn about your patient

Don't Do This

Pantomime to communicate

Rely on unapproved family members

Assume silence means agreement

Fail to read verbal and non-verbal clues

Interrupt a non-fluent patient

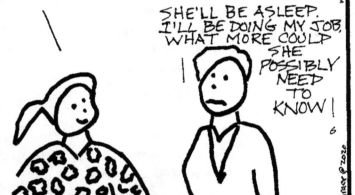

25

Informed Consent

IN THIS CHAPTER

Patients learn they have a legal right to be informed by their doctor of the procedure, alternatives and risks.

Nurses are reminded of their limited role in obtaining informed consent which generally involves securing the patient's signature on the consent documents confirming the doctor and patient have engaged in the required interactive process.

Doctors learn best practices to fulfill their fiduciary obligations to patients and how best to document their actions.

Informed consent is one of the most important concepts in the world of medical malpractice law. It is one of the most frequently raised allegations against doctors because it is one of the easiest claims to prove. Think of it as the low hanging fruit in the orchard of the plaintiff's medical malpractice attorney.

When the plaintiff-patient alleges professional negligence, he is claiming there was a breach of the standard of care. In other words, a failure to do what a reasonable doctor would do under similar circumstances. Because technical medical issues are almost always involved, expert testimony is generally required to assist the jury. However, the plaintiff does not need an expert witness to prove lack of informed consent. The essence of the informed consent claim is what a reasonable person would want to be told about the potential risks of the procedure. This is a concept any lay person can understand without the help of an expert. As the courts have said: "One doesn't need a weatherman to know it's raining outside."

And unlike medical negligence where the plaintiff must prove the breach of the standard of care actually caused injury, no proof of negligently caused harm is needed to establish a claim for lack of informed consent. All the plaintiff need prove is an undisclosed complication occurred and had he known he never would have consented nor would a reasonable person do so. Thus, a technically perfect surgery can be the basis of a successful informed consent claim merely because a known but undisclosed complication occurred which can happen in even the most competent surgeon's hands. No wonder plaintiffs and their lawyers love this theory of legal liability!

In all states, a patient's consent to a medical procedure must be informed.[44] Legally, a patient can only give his informed consent if the doctor has adequately explained the proposed treatment or procedure in language he can understand. In most states, this means the likely success of the proposed treatment or procedure, the risks and benefits, and the alternatives. The focus of the law is on disclosure of material substantial risks any reasonable person would want to know in deciding how to proceed, rather than mere minor risks.

Here are the essentials doctors and nurses need to keep in mind:

- The obtaining of a patient's valid legal consent requires an *interactive process* between doctor and patient. This means the patient must be free to ask questions and receive answers to all his questions.
- The doctor has a *non-delegable duty* which arises from his personal fiduciary relationship with the patient. In other words, the doctor may NOT legally hand off this responsibility to his nurse or other office staff members. They may be involved in the process but not to the exclusion of the doctor. For example, they may show the patient a pre-surgical video or obtain signatures on needed documents.
- The required physician disclosure of alternatives must include doing nothing. It is the right of the patient to decide to undergo the recommended procedure or no procedure at all.
- The patient's consent can be revoked at any time, including the day of surgery. It is not uncommon for patients who have previously consented to get

---

[44] American Society for Healthcare Risk Management (ASHRM), *Informed Consent and the Law*, Chicago: American Society for Healthcare Risk Management, 2000

cold feet. They may want to ask more questions for reassurance or cancel the scheduled procedure altogether.

- Informed consent is NOT a document. It is the give and take process between doctor and patient which is then evidenced by the patient's signature on a consent form.

- The physician should document the informed consent discussion in the medical record. This can be in an office note or a hospital progress note. Best practice at a minimum is to state the following: "The procedure, alternatives, and risks were discussed with the patient. All questions were answered and the patient elected to proceed." If the surgery is unusual or carries serious risks such as death or incapacity, best practice is also to include that reference in your written notes. But do not attempt to identify in writing each and every one of the potential risks you discussed. As a defense attorney many times I saw 'Murphy's Law" in action where the actual surgical complication was inadvertently omitted from the documented laundry list of potential complications. The lawsuits then focused on a swearing contest between doctor and patient whether or not that particular complication was discussed.

- The doctor should NOT document the informed consent discussion in the Operative Note. Proper informed consent occurs well before surgery. Documentation after surgery has begun will look self-serving and not believable especially if the doctor is simultaneously referencing a surgical complication.

- An informed consent requires full participation by the patient. Don't attempt to engage in the interactive process while the patient is under the influence of medication which can impair the ability to reason or communicate.

- The Joint Commission requires hospitals to utilize separate "consent to surgical/special procedures" and "consent to anesthesia" forms. These forms MUST be signed by the patient prior to the event and, if necessary, witnessed by a foreign language translator. There is a place at the end of the document for a "physician certification" that the informed consent process was completed. Best practice is to customize your own documentation as noted above rather than relying on the boilerplate language in the form.

- Nurses typically are charged with obtaining the required signatures. However, the nurse is NOT doing the informed consent process. Rather, the nurse is merely confirming with the patient the doctor has already engaged in the interactive process. The nurse is not there to answer additional patient questions about the surgery. All such questions need to be referred back to the doctor who then needs to document the subsequent conversation.

- As the "consent to anesthesia" hospital form suggests, the anesthesiologist has the same legal obligation as the surgeon to engage in the interactive informed consent process irrespective of type of anesthetic agent or mode of administration.
- If a patient is scheduled for more than one surgical procedure, the entire interactive and document process must be repeated.
- Doctors who obtain consent for one procedure but then do a completely different procedure can expect to be sued for the intentional tort of medical battery. This carries potentially graver risks in terms of punitive damages which are not insurable. The emphasis is on a substantially different surgery; for example, operating on the wrong leg, not merely converting an arthroscopic procedure on the correct leg into an open procedure.
- In addition to surgery, special procedures, and anesthesia, there are other situations where most state laws and hospital regulations require an informed consent process. These typically include: blood transfusions, HIV blood tests, bilateral tubal ligations, hysterectomies or other sterilization procedures, use of investigative drugs or devices, and human experimentation, among others.
- There is a well-recognized exception to the foregoing for true medical emergencies. When a patient lacks capacity to consent and a surrogate decision-maker cannot be found and treatment is immediately necessary to prevent death or serious injury, medical care may proceed.

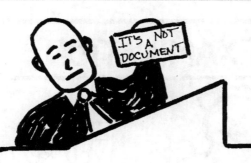

Do This

Know it's common to be sued for lack of consent

Explain the procedure, alternatives, and risks

Engage in an interactive process

Document the discussion

Repeat as necessary until the patient decides

Don't Do This

Assume a written document is the consent

Delegate the interactive process to another

Conduct the process with a medicated patient

Document the discussion in the Op Note

Become angry if the patient revokes consent

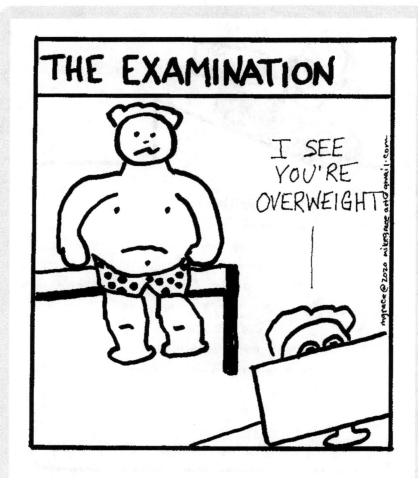

26
Conduct During Examinations

IN THIS CHAPTER

Patients recognize situations during physical examinations where their modesty and dignity are ignored without explanation.

Nurses, and particularly doctors, are reminded to empathize with their patients' needs and wishes during physical examinations.

What healthcare providers say and do during examinations might be more amusing if the roles were reversed. One suspects things would proceed a bit differently if the doctor were disrobed while the patient remained clothed! Misunderstandings can easily arise during physical examinations especially if the provider is insensitive to patient modesty and dignity.[45]

No woman enjoys being put in stirrups. Being left there exposed by the medical assistant who departs with the promise to get the doctor is seldom appreciated. Especially since the doctor never seems to arrive quickly! The loud and clear non-verbal message is a disregard for the patient's dignity. Would it have been inconvenient for the gowned patient to sit demurely awaiting the doctor's arrival?

As a medical malpractice defense attorney, I represented scores of obstetricians over the years. One of the more memorable clients kept leaving the

---

[45] North Carolina Medical Board, Guidelines for Avoiding Misunderstandings During Patient Encounters and Physical Examinations, 1991, Amended Mar 2019, https://www.ncmedboard.org/resources-information/professional-resources/laws-rules-position-statements/position-statements/guidelines_for_avoiding

patient in the stirrups in the middle of a prolonged difficult delivery to answer his cell phone. The calls were not medical emergencies. It turned out it was his birthday and he was planning his own party!

Doctors need to explain to patients what they propose to do during the exam before doing it. I was once hired to defend a gynecologist's conduct during a breast examination. The patient was sitting on the edge of the exam table wearing only a paper gown. Silently the doctor entered the room. Without warning, he ripped open the front of the paper gown, and grabbed her breasts with both hands. The startled patient screamed! Predictably a lawsuit for assault and emotional distress ensued.

Conduct of pelvic exams is a frequent source of misunderstanding and litigation. Ob-gyns, internists, and general practitioners all need to take the time to explain to their patients what will be involved in the examination. Especially if the woman has a particular pelvic history likely requiring more time for evaluation. Many lawsuits have been filed by women who decided: "His hand was inside me too long. He was obviously enjoying himself!"

Less frequent but equally problematic is the prolonged prostate exam. One family practitioner, without explanation, was insistent his protesting patient kneel on all fours on top of the exam table during the prostate exam—while his female assistant observed!

Much more common are examples of unanesthetized or inadequately anesthetized patients who complain of pain and insist the doctor stop the elective procedure or examination. If a conscious patient denies having received an anesthetic before a colon examination, believe him! Take the time to check the medical record. If a patient complains of excruciating pain during a procedure such as insertion of a pressurized catheter in his femoral artery and demands it be stopped, stop the procedure or administer more anesthetic if the patient is agreeable. Just because a patient agreed to the procedure and it has commenced does not mean the doctor can override the patient's demand to cease.

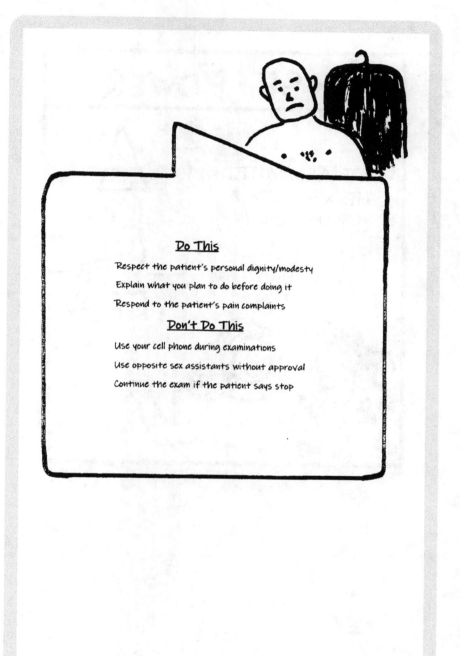

Do This

Respect the patient's personal dignity/modesty

Explain what you plan to do before doing it

Respond to the patient's pain complaints

Don't Do This

Use your cell phone during examinations

Use opposite sex assistants without approval

Continue the exam if the patient says stop

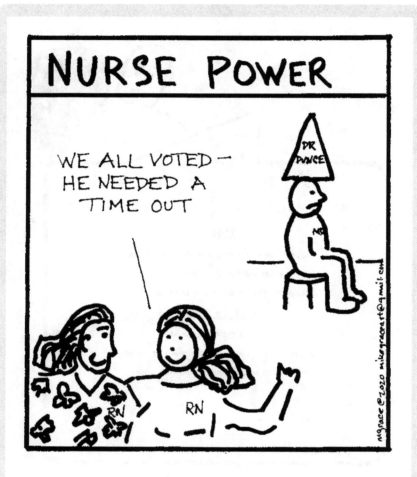

27
Communicating in the Medical Record

IN THIS CHAPTER

Patients learn their medical record is a legal document, the accuracy of which is key to proper diagnosis and treatment.

Nurses and doctors are reminded about proper charting techniques and the pitfalls of cut and paste short-cuts.

Proper documentation in a patient's medical record, whether handwritten or electronic, operates by fundamentally different rules than verbal and non-verbal expression. Writings are permanent and can be read and reread for comprehension. They are a future reference when memories fade about what transpired when facts were fresher. They are more laborious by nature than the quickly spoken word and can therefore be polished for more precise clarity. But unlike telephonic and face-to-face communication, writings lack immediacy as well as real-time feedback. Unpacking the meaning of the written word is not assisted by questions, tone of voice, facial expression, or body language. If words are not carefully chosen, the risk of miscommunication is heightened.

The patient's medical record is a legal document. Life and death decisions may be made based on its contents. Earlier documented tests and treatments become building blocks for future decision-making. Creating an entry in the patient's medical record is truly a time "to say what you mean and mean what you say." The entry should be accurate and complete. As all healthcare providers have been taught: "Not charted, not done." The medical record will be used by risk managers investigating an incident, by state and federal officials responding to a complaint, and by attorneys litigating fault.[46]

The medical record is used by a provider in solo practice to speak to himself (for later reference) as well as the patient's other current and future providers who obtain copies. The sole practitioner is also speaking to health plans, employers where there is a workers' compensation claim, and third parties who lawfully subpoena the records.

The hospital medical record is written for a similar but much wider audience—other doctors and nurses simultaneously caring for the patient. As we have seen, there is seldom a continuity of hospitalist providers during a patient's hospital stay. However, while the doctors may change, the medical record provides a continuity of care. Each subsequent hospitalist should be aware of what her predecessors have done and why. Likewise, nurses chart throughout the shift about the patient's condition. Future shifts refer back to and rely upon the nursing record.

Here are the guideposts all creators of medical records need to keep in mind:

- While of vital importance, documentation in the medical record is not a substitute for the provider talking to the patient or one another.
- An electronic trail is automatically made anytime anyone enters an electronic medical record. The trail identifies the person, the time and the date, as well as any notes or changes made. There is no such thing as anonymity.
- Changes can be made by the same provider to his own earlier notes. However, the original entry as well as the corrected version are retrievable. Nothing ever truly disappears.
- Changes cannot be made by a provider to someone else's documentation.
- Documentation should be made contemporaneously as events occur or as soon as practicable thereafter. Charting days later is never as accurate because memories begin to fade.
- Don't forget to document all phone conversations with the patient and other providers including the date and time.

---

[46] Gaffey, A., Groves, S., "The Clinical Record," In Carroll, R. (ed) *Risk Management Handbook for Healthcare Organizations*, 6th edition, 2011: 331–365

- Medical record charting needs to be kept factual and limited to information within the first-hand knowledge of the person making the notation. The record should never be used for speculation, rumors, or unverified information. Nor should the record be used for a back-and-forth debate between colleagues.
- Proofread the accuracy of your entries including spelling and grammar. This is especially critical if the entry was made using dictation systems or voice recognition software. Your entries in the medical record will be key pieces of evidence in any litigation and sloppy entries will be used by clever attorneys to undermine your credibility. No healthcare provider wants to see an embarrassing medical record blown up big as a barn in the courtroom for public derision.
- A huge problem with the use of electronic medical records is the ability in most systems to cut and paste language from the reports of others. Doctors and nurses in a rush often use this poor practice when they adopt and disseminate information not of their first-hand knowledge.
- For doctors, this bad habit often appears in the cutting and pasting of the patient's medical history. Inaccurate information about a patient keeps getting passed along from one provider to the next, all blithely unaware the information isn't true. Don't think the sloppy inaccuracies will go unnoticed. With increasing reliance on patient portals, for the first time many patients are now actually reading what has been written about them.
- For nurses, cutting and pasting often happens with Braden scoring for the development of pressure ulcers. Skin breakdown in hospitalized patients can occur within hours. Braden scoring was designed to evaluate rapid skin changes based on factors such as sensory perception, mobility and nutrition. Busy nurses often don't take the time to do their own scoring and adopt the score from the prior shift. "Suddenly" the patient has a severe skin breakdown which must be reported to governmental authorities for investigation.
- Opinions should only be expressed by those persons qualified to render an opinion. For instance, physician specialists called to evaluate a patient are typically asked to provide an opinion within their own field of expertise in an evaluation report. They should not venture out of their "swim lane" by offering conjecture better left to other specialists.
- Nurses should not express opinions about the medical care or clinical judgment of physicians. They need to confine themselves to nursing matters within their own specialty.

- An adverse patient event should be documented in an incident report. These are special types of legal documents afforded particular protections under the law. They are used by hospital risk managers and others to investigate events and, where appropriate, develop corrective action plans. Copies of the incident report should never be put in the patient's medical record.

- However, all patient care should be carefully documented in the medical record. For example, a patient's fall in the bathroom should be included in the medical record as a factual occurrence. The entry should state when the fall occurred, who responded, and how quickly. Any statements by the patient should be put in quotation marks such as "I had to pee and didn't have time to ring for the nurse." The physical assessment and any injuries should be detailed and any treatment described. For example: "The patient sustained a bruise to his left forearm and a 2 centimeter skin tear on his left knee which was bandaged. Dr. Mark Russo was notified." However, there should be no statement in the medical record about the cause of the fall or opinions about blame. That should be left for the investigation of the incident report.

- The patient's medical record should never be used for personnel or employment matters. For example, if two nurses get into a disagreement about a patient's care, that matter should be documented elsewhere such as a report to Human Resources.

- The rules for communication in a paper (non-electronic) chart are largely the same with a few caveats. Late entries should be clearly labeled, dated, timed and signed. Changes to the paper record should be done with a simple line through the inaccuracy so it is still legible, followed by the new dated, timed, and initialed entry.

- Keep in mind there is no such thing as getting away with a forgery or alteration of the record. Handwriting experts have sophisticated equipment at their disposal to analyze documents. Even the ink in pens is coded by year to thwart unsuspecting forgers!

I once defended a cardiologist who was sued, along with the cardiac surgeon and hospital, for wrongful death of a patient during surgery. The allegation against my client was inappropriate dosage of a cardiac medication. The defense handwriting expert proved to the jury that my client had not made the decimal point in question. The entire case turned on a single ink dot in a handwritten medical record! The jury learned a family member of the deceased patient worked in the hospital, got access to the medical record, and added the decimal point himself!

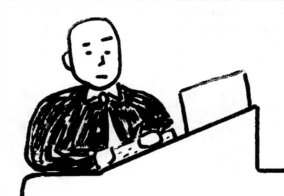

Do This

Recognize medical records are legal documents

Chart only factual, first-hand information

Make entries contemporaneously with events

Confine opinions to your specialty

Follow "late entry" and correction protocols

Don't Do This

Cut and paste other's work if unverified

Express criticism, fault or blame

Attempt to change or correct another's note

Put an Incident Report in the patient's chart

Attempt to alter or forge a document

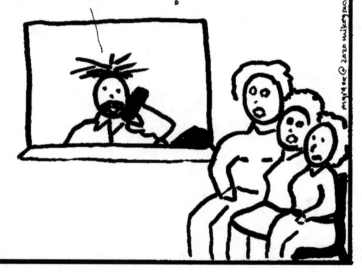

28
Confidentiality

IN THIS CHAPTER

Patients learn about the scope and limits of the confidentiality of their medical conversations and documents.

Nurses and doctors are reminded about the practical aspects of HIPAA and the consequences of violating its provisions.

Doctors are reminded they are legally responsible for breaches of patient confidentiality by their employees.

There are two important types of patient confidentiality for all healthcare workers to know about—verbal exchanges between doctor and patient under state law and protected health information (PHI) under federal law.

The shield of confidentiality of doctor-patient verbal communication has long been recognized in the laws of all fifty states. But like other well-known legally protected speech (such as between a priest and penitent or between a married couple), there are some important exceptions. A doctor may not keep confidential any statement by a patient of his intent to harm himself or another person. For instance, telling your psychiatrist you plan to kill your cheating husband must be disclosed for the protection of the third party. Most states don't protect verbal communication between patient and nurse or other office staff unless they were physically present during the verbal exchange with the doctor. And, like all state communication privileges, the privilege can be waived, but only by the patient, not the doctor.

By far the most dynamic of the confidentiality laws is found in the Health Insurance Portability and Accountability Act enacted by Congress almost thirty years ago.[47] HIPAA changed how the business of American healthcare treated patient confidentiality and provided a national framework of consumer protections. HIPAA has two major components—security protections for health data and privacy rules for patients. Our focus is on privacy because it impacts all healthcare provider communication.

HIPAA governs what "covered entities" may do with "protected health information" (PHI). Covered entities include all healthcare plans, healthcare organizations, hospitals, and healthcare workers. It does *not* prevent other persons or entities like family members or employers from disseminating your health information. Protected health information includes individually identifiable information about past, present, or future health status. PHI can be unlawfully disseminated either verbally or in writing. Stiff civil and criminal penalties attach for each breach of PHI by a covered entity. Doctors and hospitals beware—you are legally responsible for HIPAA violations committed by your employees acting in the scope and course of their employment. Training employed staff is therefore critically important.

HIPAA is complex and its rules are constantly reinterpreted and refined by the U.S. Department of Health and Human Services (HHSS). Consultation with an attorney and review of the law is always recommended. However, here are some of the more enduring practical aspects of HIPAA which all healthcare providers should know:

- The only persons authorized by law to access a patient's PHI include the patient, his authorized personal representative, and the treating healthcare providers. Treating providers may also send copies to other healthcare providers or plans but only as needed for treatment or payment.
- In Chapter 20 we discussed patient authorization for PHI to be shared with family members. By the same process, a patient can also authorize friends or significant others to receive his protected health information.
- If you are not caring for a patient you have no right to "peek" into the medical records. Remember, electronic medical records keep a digital trail of anyone who accesses the record, even if no new entry to the record is made.

---

[47] The Health Insurance Portability and Accountability Act (HIPAA) of 1996, https://www.hhs.gov/ocr/hipaa

As the hospital Risk Manager, I investigated the case of an older doctor who couldn't resist keeping tabs on his younger estranged boyfriend by repeatedly accessing his medical record. The patient's suspicions were confirmed by a hospital audit which revealed multiple occasions over many months when the jealous jilted doctor entered the electronic system. Suffice it to say his standing with the California Medical Board was permanently damaged!

- Accessing a medical record and selling the information will get your medical or nursing license revoked. Unfortunately, there have been a few cases of healthcare workers accessing a hospitalized celebrity's records for the purpose of selling the data to the tabloid press.
- Healthcare professionals are never permitted to share the identity of their patients on social media no matter how tempting to be the "person in-the-know" about the identity of the drunk driver who was brought into the emergency department the night before.
- Hospital receptionists are not even allowed to acknowledge a particular person is in the facility receiving treatment. This can be difficult where the call purports to come from an out-of-state family member sincerely worried about their loved one's condition. Refer the call to the hospital risk manager who will likely explain the privacy purpose of the law, not confirm if the patient is present, and obtain the family member's contact information. Then, if the patient consents, a call back about the patient's health status can occur.
- However, so-called "incidental" disclosures of limited information may be allowed. For example, a front desk staff person may call "Ruth" or "Mrs. Weinstein" from the waiting room to see the doctor so long as no information about diagnosis or treatment is mentioned. And the full name of a patient displayed in his hospital room is also considered an "incidental" disclosure.
- Nurses should never enter a patient's hospital room announcing administration of a specific medication if there are third parties present. Drug names are frequently associated with a medical diagnosis even by lay people.
- All healthcare workers need to be cognizant of patient privacy in public places like hallways and elevators. Referring to a patient by hospital room number when discussing diagnosis or treatment is a breach of PHI even if the patient name is not used because anyone within earshot can figure out the identity of the patient.

- Doctors may email patients about their medical condition—but only through secure servers. Encryption software is required and best practice is to use "patient portals" established by most healthcare delivery systems.
- No healthcare provider should put PHI or identifiable patient photos on his mobile phone or unencrypted laptop computer. The data on such devices is not secure. Electronic devices are lost and stolen all the time. If a lost or stolen device contains such information, elaborate procedures about patient notification and remedial action are triggered by HIPAA's security rules.

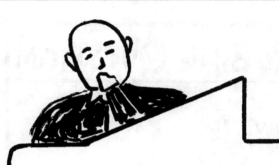

Do This

Remember only treating providers may access PMI

Remember electronic records have digital trails

Protect patient confidentiality in public places

Use patient portals and encryption to communicate

Don't Do This

Post patient names or photos on social media

Acknowledge who is receiving treatment

Use patient room numbers with diagnoses

Identify patient medications to 3rd parties

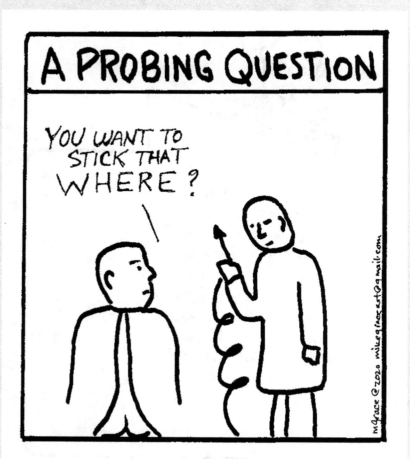

29
Sex Talk

IN THIS CHAPTER

Patients are encouraged to initiate the conversation with their healthcare provider about any sexual concerns.

Nurses, and particularly doctors, need to be comfortable talking about sexual matters, especially testing, and to understand the special laws governing treatment of minors.

Sexual health is too important to be ignored by healthcare professionals. It is not a time for wrong-headed assumptions. Healthcare providers shouldn't think a patient with a sexual problem will automatically bring it up without prompting. And patients shouldn't operate under the misimpression "if it were important the doctor would have asked."

Fortunately, talking about sex is getting easier for most people. Perhaps we're taking our cue from television. Pharmaceutical advertisements for erectile dysfunction (ED) and vaginal itching (VI) compete in prime time with cucumber graphics about Peyronie's Disease (PD) and the plethora of sexually transmitted diseases (STDs).

In particular, all doctors need to be comfortable talking about sexual testing. If the doctor doesn't initiate the conversation, the testing often does not occur. For instance, all doctors should ask their patients if they have had an HIV test. Clinical data shows one of the largest barriers to widespread community HIV testing programs is the doctor's reticence to bring up the subject. A poster on the waiting room wall is not sufficient. Older practitioners, in particular, may need education. Knowing who should be tested and why, as well as techniques for broaching the subject with patients, increase provider compliance with testing programs.[48] Even married middle aged heterosexual women may benefit from HIV testing!

If the doctor is not at ease talking about sex, the patient won't be either. All doctors need to ask sexually pertinent questions without embarrassment or judgment, expressed or implied. And for the reluctant patient, the doctor needs to be prepared to explain why the information is important to assess the patient's health.

Unfortunately, some doctors and their staffs still allow their personal biases to impact patient care. One middle aged male patient requested his long-time Midwestern primary care physician for an HIV test. The doctor refused saying: "No. I'm not ordering that. You don't need it." "Yes, I think I do," insisted the patient. "What? You're not telling me you're queer, are you?" The embarrassed patient reluctantly responded, "Well, actually I am." The disgusted doctor ordered the test but a palpable chill descended on the doctor and his normally friendly staff. The patient ended their decade long relationship and changed providers.

A discussion of "sex talk" would not be complete without a reference to teenage sexuality. Medical treatment of minors is a special subject with rules varying considerably from state to state.[49] However, in general minors lack the legal capacity to consent to medical treatment *except* in matters of sexual health. And in most states, this sexually related treatment is confidential without parental knowledge or involvement. For example, minors can receive forms of birth control, pregnancy care, and treatment for STDs without mom or dad being the wiser. (However, a minor's insistence on sterilization is universally disallowed.) The doctor is bound by the laws of confidentiality and cannot share the fact or details with the minor's parents without the minor's permission.

As we've discussed in Chapter 18, young people may be reluctant to speak candidly with a doctor about "personal" matters. It is up to the provider to read the situation and proceed accordingly.

---

[48] Rizza, S., MacGowan, R., et al., "HIV Screening in the Health Care Setting: Status, Barriers, and Potential Solutions," Symposium on Antimicrobial Therapy, 2012 Sept 1; 87(9): 1–34

[49] National District Attorneys' Association, *Minor Consent to Medical Treatment Laws*, 2013

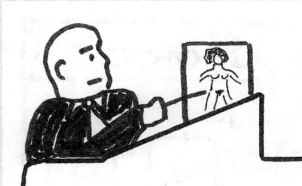

Do This

Be at ease talking about sexual health

Raise the subject of sexual testing

Know why sexual testing is important for all

Honor a patient's request for sexual testing

Don't Do This

Make assumptions about sexual problems

Wait for the patient to raise sexual health

Allow personal biases to affect professional relations

Seek parental consent to treat minors

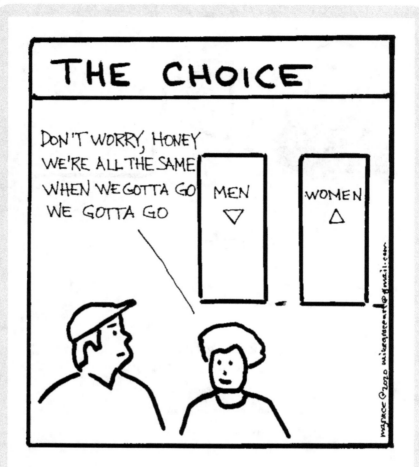

30

The Transgender and
Non-Binary Patient

IN THIS CHAPTER

Patients, nurses, and doctors are presented with best communication practices with transgender and non-binary patients recognizing the need for education within the entire medical team.

In our rapidly changing world, healthcare providers are now encountering more patients who are transgender or identify as neither male nor female. The term "transgender" refers to people whose gender identity does not coincide with the sex assigned at birth. The term "non-binary" is an imprecise umbrella term which has been used to describe persons who are gender fluid or who reject the concept of gender.[50]

The transgender and non-binary patient should be afforded the same rights of healthcare access and respectful medical treatment as binary patients. While the federal regulation implementing the "gender identity" non-discrimination provision of the Affordable Care Act is currently under constitutional challenge in the federal courts,[51] The Joint Commission and many medical professional

---

[50] The University of Iowa Healthcare, "Quick tips for medical providers of transgender patients-The Transcare approach," https://www.uihc.org/health-topics/quick-tips-medical-providers-transgender-patients

[51] Steuer, K., Davis, K., "Respecting Gender Identity in Healthcare: Regulatory Requirements and Recommendations for Treating Transgender Patients," The Health Lawyer, 2017 Feb; 29(3): 1, 3–9, https://www.americanbar.org/groups/gpsolo/publications/gpsolo_ereport/2017/respecting_gender_identity_healthcare_regulatory_requirements

associations have specifically endorsed the rights of the transgender and gender diverse communities.[52]

This expanding patient population presents challenges and opportunities for improved provider-patient communication and treatment. In 2015, over 27,000 transgender persons across the country participated in the U.S. Transgender Survey which highlighted the patterns of discrimination across society. The most common barriers to receiving healthcare were lack of insurance coverage, mistreatment by healthcare providers, and providers' discomfort and lack of experience working with and treating transgender patients.[53]

Working appropriately with this special population takes education, training, and practice—not just by clinicians but by their office staff as well. Here are the basics to keep in mind:

- We all need to learn the same vocabulary in order to communicate effectively and avoid embarrassment. Here's a brief glossary of additional terms:
  Sexual orientation—sexual identity in relation to gender(s) to which a person is attracted
  Gender identity—a personal conception of oneself as male/female or neither
  Gender expression—the external display of gender by name, pronouns, or appearance
  Trans Man—used for a person assigned female at birth, but identifies and lives as a man
  Trans Woman—assigned as a male at birth, but identifies and lives as a woman
  Cisgender—a person whose gender identity coincides with the sex assigned at birth
- When a patient calls to make an appointment and identifies as trans or non-binary, the staff member should ask the name the patient wants to be called by in the office as well as what pronouns the patient prefers. Staff should also explain for insurance billing purposes it will be necessary to know if any other names appear on legal documents.

---

[52] Kelly, M., Providing Transgender and Non-Binary Care at Planned Parenthood, 2018; 28 (citing documents from The American Academy of Pediatrics, American Academy of Physician Assistants, The American College of Obstetricians and Gynecologists (ACOG), The American Medical Association, The American Psychological Association, The American Public Health Association, and The Endocrine Society)

[53] Kelly, M., Providing Transgender and Non-Binary Care at Planned Parenthood, 2018; 41–43

- Preferred pronouns can include male (he, him, his), female (she, her, hers), or non-binary (they, them, theirs or ze, zim, zirs or sie, hir, hirs).
- When the patient arrives in the office, staff should ask "How would you like me to address you? What pronouns do you prefer?"
- Try to avoid titles like Mister, Missus, Miss, or Miz until the patient has clarified a preference.
- Be sensitive to the fact most patients will not want their status revealed in public places. Remember, transgender persons are often the victim of violence and discrimination. As comic and social commentator Trevor Noah reminds us: "Just because it's not happening to you doesn't mean it's not happening."
- Don't worry about making a mistake with the name or pronoun. This is new territory for most people. Quietly acknowledge the mistake, apologize and move on. "Sorry, I realized I called you by the wrong name."
- Office forms should provide non-binary gender identification options, preferably space for the patient to describe themselves rather than checking boxes. This information should then be made available to the entire office staff in the electronic record.
- Just as with the office staff, doctor and nurse providers should also clarify in an initial meeting how the patient prefers to be addressed. Make a note in the chart and use that name for all future encounters. People should be given the respect of being called the name they prefer.
- Clinicians should avoid idle curiosity about genital status unless pertinent to medical care.
- No one in the office should refer to the patient as "it" or "the transgender one." Obviously, no derogatory term or description is appropriate in a culturally sensitive healthcare environment. This includes negative facial reactions and body language.
- As with all patients, confidentiality is paramount.

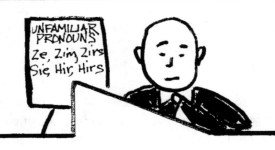

Do This

Provide equal access to medical care

Provide respectful culturally sensitive care

Call patients by their name of choice

Apologize if you use the wrong name

Use patient preference pronouns

Don't Do This

Publicly "out" trans or non-binary patients

Objectify trans or non-binary patients

Use derogatory words or non-verbal actions

Use formal titles like "Mr." until clarified

Fail to educate staff

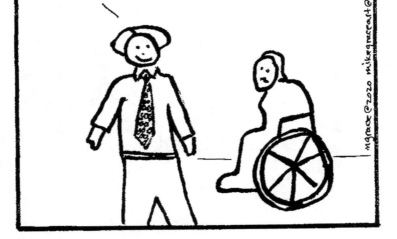

31

The Elderly Patient

IN THIS CHAPTER

Patients, nurses, and doctors learn about communicating with the elderly population and suggested strategies for taking into account their special needs.

Talking with the elderly patient can be an especially rewarding experience. These survivors of depressions and world wars have also been witnesses to mind-boggling technological changes. They are our society's long-distance runners and we have much to learn from them. If we take the time.

Interpersonal communication with our older citizens is like talking with anyone else, only a bit different.[54] In essence, it requires more patience, a heightened awareness of any cognitive or sensory deficits, and a slower pace. It is wise to keep in mind the observation of philosopher and writer C.S. Lewis: "How incessant and great are the ills with which a prolonged old age is replete."

Here are some best practices for all healthcare professionals to follow:

- Don't rush the patient. Everything takes them a little longer including walking, sitting down, getting up, and processing information.
- Show respect for the patient's age and status. Honor the patient with the courtesy he is due.

---

[54] Robinson, T., "Improving Communication With Older Patients: Tips From the Literature," Fam Pract Manag, (2006 Sep); 13(8): 73–78

- Introduce the patient to your staff. She will feel more comfortable knowing who she is dealing with. And remember future "re-introductions" may be needed. "Mrs. Novak, you remember my medical assistant, James. He'll be happy to show you to the restroom." Mentioning the name refreshes recollection and can spare the patient the embarrassment of having to ask.
- Take a personal interest. "Tell me about yourself." "Where did you grow up?" "How do you spend your time?" Elderly patients grew up without electronic diversions when people talked more to one another. Take the time to know the patient and you'll have a more memorable and satisfying relationship.
- Don't interrupt. Listen to what the patient says, both the words and the meaning behind the words. Consider the tone of voice and body language. Look for changes in the patient's condition which can occur rapidly with advancing age. Also listen for signs of depression and loneliness which often afflict the elderly.
- Be ready to probe the truthfulness of responses such as "I'm fine" and "As good as can be expected at my age." Older patients tend to be stoic. Vague statements of wellbeing may mask a more serious situation.
- Always reconcile the patient's medication list. Older people typically take more medicine, often prescribed by different providers. And older patients tend to react more strongly to medication than younger people. Consider the individual and synergistic effects of all medication, especially on memory, cognition, and motor skills. For example, the risk for falls increases when the older person is taking more than four medications and certain types of drugs.[55]
- Speak more slowly than normal. Rapid speech is more difficult to process.
- Use shorter sentences and avoid jargon and long monologues. Also emphasize any shift in topic or time frame.
- Speak up but, of course, don't shout. If the patient has a suspected hearing loss, encourage the patient to keep the referral appointment to a specialist for a hearing test.
- Sit on the same level as the patient. And face the patient. It is easier for them to hear and read your facial expression. And don't cover your mouth with your hands. The older patient may rely somewhat on lip reading to process what you say.

---

[55] Weiss, C., "Fall Prevention Among the Elderly," Nursing Spectrum.com, 2002 June

- Verify the patient has an Advance Directive for Healthcare and that you have a copy in the chart. Also confirm who the patient authorized to know his personal health information and document the conversation.
- Pay particular attention to the concerns of "approved" family members who may accompany the patient. With advancing age, you are likely to be dealing with them a lot in the future. Including them in treatment plans is essential, especially if they are involved as actual caregivers. Satisfy yourself the "team" is all on the same page—you, the patient, and the involved family members.
- As with all patients but even more critical with the elderly, use feedback loops to ensure the Receiver has understood the Message you've sent. Ask the elderly patient to repeat back what she is to do.
- The use of written, easily read materials is also helpful. Review discharge instructions with the patient and use a highlighter to emphasize key sections.

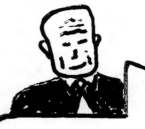

Do This

Show respect for the patient's age and status

Take the time to show a personal interest

Always update the medication list

Speak slowly while facing the patient

Include approved family members

Don't Do This

Rush or interrupt the patient

Ignore evaluation of potential mental decline

Assume the truth of stoic health responses

Mumble or cover your mouth when speaking

Ignore opinions of caregivers

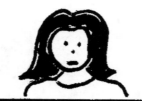
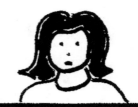

32

The Seriously Ill Patient

IN THIS CHAPTER

Patients, nurses, and doctors learn communicating with a very ill or dying patient presents unique challenges requiring extra patience, sensitivity, and clarity.

The sicker the patient, the more impediments exist preventing him from receiving the Message intended by the Sender. And the graver the illness, the more important the Message be understood. This is the conundrum of communicating with the seriously ill patient.

Think of the barriers identified in Chapter 8—bias, health illiteracy, white coat stress, pain, medication effects, memory impairment, sensory loss, language, cultural confusion, fear of treatment, and terror of death and dying—as being on growth hormones. The involved healthcare team can expect a near constant battle to break through these over-sized obstacles. Just as the "success" of understanding is achieved one day, the patient can "backslide" the next. The watchwords are patience and perseverance.

For many patients the mere mention of the word "cancer" is tantamount to a death sentence. Such an ingrained core belief is often more emotional than logical. And logic never trumps emotion.

These patients may proceed through the well-documented five stages of grief—emotions of denial, anger, bargaining, depression and acceptance. While there is no empirical proof most people experience these emotions, much less in the linear order originally described by Elizabeth Kubler-Ross, it is useful for healthcare professionals to keep in mind the emotional mindset of the seriously ill patient can shift from encounter to encounter.[56] The ebb and flow of emotions is natural. Don't try to cheer them up or talk them down; "just ride the waves of emotion with them."[57]

Here are some best practices when talking with the seriously ill patient:

- If you are reporting bad news, consider this step-by-step template: sit down, mention the purpose of the meeting, foreshadow the bad news, speak directly and unequivocally, remain quiet while the patient absorbs the news, ask what the patient knows about the disease, demonstrate empathy, and make a plan for the next steps.[58]
- Always encourage the patient to express his feelings without interruption.
- Encourage note-taking as a tool to remember what has been discussed and for topics the patient wants to raise.
- Encourage the involvement of caring friends and family members during doctor-patient visits. They can not only lend emotional support but serve as resources to the patient after the encounter about what was said.
- Be compassionate and caring. But don't patronize the patient with well-meaning expressions such as "I know just how you feel."
- Be mindful of your own mood and affect. All patients, but especially the most vulnerable, may pick up emotional cues from the healthcare provider. There is a reason some of the most upbeat doctors work with the sickest patients. Oncologists are notorious for their cheerful dispositions!
- Don't invade the patient's personal space without first asking permission. "May I give you a hug?" While author A.A. Milne's Winnie the Pooh correctly recognized "a hug is always the right size," an unexpected embrace could be upsetting or even physically painful.
- The sickest patients tend to be treated by teams of doctor specialists. This requires more effort on the part of each doctor to communicate clearly with every other doctor, both verbally and in the written record. More doctors also mean more medications to reconcile on each visit.
- The sickest patients also tend to have the most complex medical conditions and treatments. Be extra careful about the "mumbo jumbo" of medical

---

[56] Gregory, C., "The Five Stages of Grief-An Examination of the Kubler-Ross Model," Psycom, https.//www.psycom.net/authors/christina-gregory-phd

[57] Riecke, P., *How to Talk with Sick, Dying, and Grieving People*, 2018: 77

[58] Headly, A., "Communication Skills: A Call for Teaching to the Test," American Journal of Medicine, 2007 Oct 1; 120(10): 910–915; https://www.amjmed.com/article/S0002-9343(07)00726-7/fulltext

lingo. Constantly read your audience for understanding of your Message. Reinforce the Message with easily understood literature and illustrations. And constantly encourage questions to assess comprehension. The more complicated the Message, the more likely it will need to be repeated to be fully absorbed.

- Optimism and hopefulness still require truthfulness. If the patient demands "to know the odds," respect those wishes. Don't ever deceive a patient. But any discussion of statistical chances of survival needs to be carefully explained. They are never a prognosticator of how any specific individual will respond to treatment. And, if the patient is receiving "new" therapy, caveats about the lack of large sample studies need to be reinforced. The human mind is powerful. No doctor wants a patient who is told he has "one year to live" to die on the 366th day.

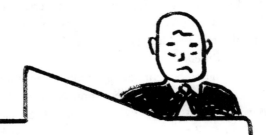

Do This

Watch for shifts in the emotional mindset

Encourage the patient to share feelings

Encourage the presence of supportive family

Encourage notetaking during visits

Speak honestly about treatment and prognosis

Don't Do This

Use the mumbo jumbo of complex medicine

Patronize with well-intended sentiments

Ignore the effect of your own mood on others

Invade personal space without permission

Become impatient with repeated questions

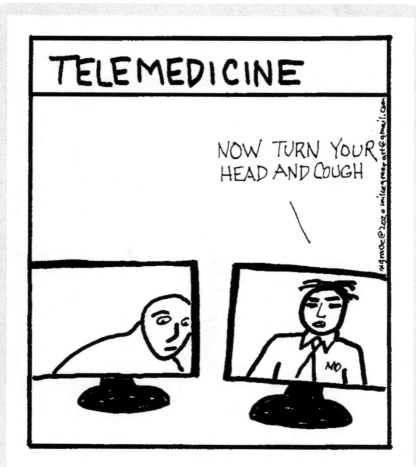

33
Telemedicine

IN THIS CHAPTER

Patients, nurses, and doctors learn to maximize the advantage of telemedicine communication by attention to issues of self-identification, environmental distraction, modeling instructions, and camera angles.

Telemedicine has been around a lot longer than most people realize with its origins in the telegraph and radio industries. However, as a visual tool it has been growing rapidly in recent years fueled by fiber optics and compressed video streaming capabilities. Now in the time of a global pandemic its medical use has quickly become mainstreamed across all specialties and geographic regions facilitated by the federal government's temporary relaxation of encryption regulations during the nationwide public health emergency. At least for the time being, private "unsecure" cell phone "face-time" applications can be used in telemedicine encounters.[59]

By definition telemedicine involves provider and patient in different locations. It can take place in formal settings designed for the purpose: for example, a physician specialist in a metropolitan hospital's conference room communicating with a patient hundreds of miles away in a remote rural clinic. More often today, the physician is using his home or work station computer to speak

---

[59] U.S. Department of Health & Human Services, "Notification of Enforcement Discretion for Telehealth Remote Communications During the COVID-19 Nationwide Public Health Emergency," https://www.hhs.gov/hipaa/for-professionals/special-topics/emergency-preparedness/notification-enforcement-discretion-telehealth/index.html

with a patient at home holding a smart phone. While both scenarios offer the same potential of more efficient and less costly healthcare, few providers and even fewer patients have been trained to communicate effectively in this situation. Here are the factors all participants—doctors, nurses, and patients—need to keep in mind:

- The physical setting must be free of visual and auditory distractions. Everyone should be aware of what is visible behind them within camera range. For example, visible spinning ceiling fans can interfere with concentration. Doors should be closed to prevent interruptions. If the patient has a television on in the background, the healthcare provider should ask the patient to turn it off so he can hear without interference.
- At the outset of the encounter, introductions need to be made with identification of the provider's name and credentials. Oftentimes patients have never previously seen or met the provider they are speaking with. The provider also needs to have the patient confirm his identity and date of birth. Finally, as part of the introduction, the provider needs to secure the patient's verbal agreement to proceed telephonically, to confirm the patient understands the encounter is not on an encrypted line if that's the case, and to advise the patient of standard "traditional" evaluation options.
- The same rules of patient privacy and confidentiality apply to telemedicine as to in-person encounters. Providers need to make sure that non-essential persons are not in the room with them. Providers also need to verify the patient is alone. If not, the provider needs to secure the patient's permission to proceed and document that fact.
- The provider should make sure his face fills the camera frame and, if necessary, instruct the patient to do the same. By its nature the camera does not display body language but well-lit facial expression is an important communicator of telemedicine Messages.
- Both parties need to be aware of the time lag between transmission of their voices. Each person needs to wait until the other has finished speaking before starting to speak themselves. Otherwise, both parties will be talking over each other compromising the understanding of both Sender and Receiver.
- The same standard of care applies to telemedicine as traditional encounters. Likewise, the same rules of ADA accommodations and informed consent also apply.

- By necessity the physical examination will require the provider's coaching and the patient's cooperation. Often the provider will need to model the behavior desired from the patient. For example, for an eye examination, tell the patient to take his index finger and pull down his eye-lid as the provider demonstrates the maneuver on himself. For an orthopedic exam, ask the patient to rotate his arm as the provider demonstrates the range of motion he wants him to mimic. The provider should make sure to instruct the patient's use of the camera as needed for him to maintain proper observation.
- If the physical examination involves disrobing, the provider needs to be particularly sensitive to the patient's feelings about being seen on camera. Give precise instructions and show respect for the patient's modesty and dignity.
- If the situation requires a provider such as a home healthcare nurse to evaluate safety in the home, the nurse needs to coach the patient to angle the camera to the areas in question. Used properly, telemedicine can be an invaluable tool for tasks such as assessing fall risks in the home of elderly patients.
- As with face-to-face encounters, use teach-back strategies to confirm the patient's understanding of the treatment plan and needed follow-up.
- Full and complete documentation of the encounter in the medical record is vital. This includes the special introductory matters mentioned above.

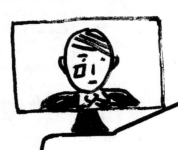

Do This

Identify yourself

Ask the patient for identification

Demonstrate examination maneuvers

Use encrypted lines whenever possible

Don't Do This

Conduct encounters with open doors

Have unnecessary colleagues present

Permit visual or auditory distractions

Forget to document informed consent

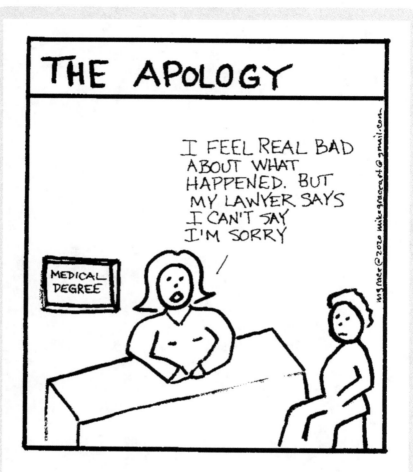

34
Doctor Disclosure and Apology

IN THIS CHAPTER

Patients learn they have a right to be informed of the occurrence of medically recognized "never" events whether occurring inside or outside of the hospital setting.

Doctors are reminded they have a legal duty of disclosure which should be done pursuant to hospital policy if the event occurred within the facility accompanied by a carefully crafted apology.

No one wants to deliver bad news and most of us are reluctant to admit we made a mistake. This vitally important topic of physician communication is where human nature collides with ethical and legal responsibilities.

There is agreement within the healthcare industry that there are certain adverse events causing death or severe injury which are largely preventable and should never occur. These adverse "never" events were first identified by federal governmental organizations after considerable research and debate almost twenty years ago. The list has grown and the National Quality Forum and the Agency for Health Research and Quality now identify twenty-nine such events.[60,61]

---

[60] National Quality Forum (NQF), *Serious Reportable Event in Healthcare—2011 Update: A Consensus Report*, Washington, DC: NQF; 2011

[61] Leapfrog, "When hospitals and surgery centers say "I'm sorry," https://www.leapfroggroup.org/influencing/never-events

Federal law and many state laws require hospitals report each occurrence to the government and the patient. The expectation is investigation and public scrutiny will improve patient safety. (Of course, patients and their health plans can never be legally charged for services associated with these adverse events.)

The twenty-nine adverse "sentinel" events fall into seven categories: surgical, product or device, patient protection, care management, environmental, radiologic, and criminal. As the saying goes: "Healthcare is a team sport" and most of these events implicate several potential actors including doctors, nurses, pharmacists, technicians, and security guards, among others. Doctors should be as familiar with the list as hospital administrators.

For the purpose of this chapter, let's focus on the adverse events in which doctors play a pivotal role. As a Risk Manager I have personally investigated almost every one of these situations. As a trial attorney I was hired to defend most of them. They may be referred to as "never" events but not because they never occur.

- Surgery (or invasive procedure) on the wrong body part or wrong patient
- Wrong surgery (or invasive procedure) performed on a patient
- Patient suicide or attempted suicide within the facility
- Patient death or serious injury from any type of medication error
- Patient death or serious injury associated with the unsafe administration of blood products
- Maternal or neonatal death or serious injury in a low-risk pregnancy
- Artificial insemination with the wrong donor sperm or egg
- Patient death or serious injury resulting from failure to follow up or communicate laboratory, pathology or radiology test results
- Patient death or serious injury resulting from electric shocks or burns

Doctors have a well-known ethical obligation "to do no harm." Patients have a legal right to their medical information. If the doctor was centrally involved in any of the adverse events enumerated above, the doctor has an ethical obligation to tell the patient.

All hospitals have written policies about disclosure of these adverse events. Most policies identify the team of persons who should be present and involved in the patient disclosure meeting including the doctor, risk manager, and senior administration officer. The policies also address the timing and manner of the planned disclosure. Doctors should not "go rogue" by ignoring the hospital's written disclosure policy. It is there for the protection of all concerned.

Sometimes the issue arises as to which doctor should be present, especially if the written policy is not explicit. In general, it should be the most involved doctor such as the attending physician or primary surgeon. If you ordered a test which was misread by radiology or the laboratory for example, you as the ordering physician should do the disclosure. Don't assume the disclosure will be done by the radiologist or pathologist who probably never met the patient.

Often there is concern about "how far" a disclosure should go. It must always be truthful and factual. Usually at the time of the disclosure meeting with the patient (or family members as appropriate), the full extent of the facts are not known and are still under investigation. There should be no speculation about where the investigation may lead. There should be no expression of blame or fault. Finger pointing will only spur criticism back at you. Oftentimes the hospital policy will encourage a statement made by the hospital administrative officer to the effect: "The hospital sincerely regrets this happened and we promise to figure out exactly how it occurred in order to prevent anything like it from ever happening again." Typically, the patient will want to be kept advised of the final result of the investigation as is his right.

These examples of "never" events which must be reported to governmental authorities are only a partial list of the kind of matters which a doctor has an obligation to disclose to his patient. By definition the twenty-nine adverse events all involve death or serious injury. However, less harmful events, whether occurring in a hospital or not, and which potentially impact a patient's health, must also be disclosed. These incidents may be similar to the twenty-nine events but non-life threatening or present a completely different type of fact pattern.

There are countless examples of possible situations requiring patient disclosure. Here are a few of the more common ones:

- Unintended harm during surgery such as nicking a nearby organ where the error is promptly recognized and repaired
- An inaccurate intra-operative sponge count leading to the immediate return of the patient to the operating room for its retrieval
- Physician administration of an incorrect medication where the error is recognized and not repeated or where a "reversal" medication was given

- The physician mistakenly orders tests, such as imaging studies, intended for another patient and the tests are performed. (Note: if the tests were only ordered and the error discovered before they were performed, there would have been no unnecessary exposure to radiation and no patient disclosure would be warranted.)

When the adverse events are not among the twenty-nine requiring hospital reporting, the physician will usually be on his own to do the disclosure since he is not governed by a hospital policy. Left to his own devices, some doctors look for the easy way out. Often as a Risk Manager I had to counsel surgeons about proper disclosures. Only mentioning the event in the operative report is not sufficient! Most patients never obtain or read their operative reports. An ethical disclosure requires direct contact so the patient's questions can be answered. As comedian Robin Williams chided: "What's right is what's left if you do everything else wrong." And, of course, this disclosure conversation should be documented in the patient's medical chart.

A proper disclosure is also in the doctor's legal interest. If he withholds information about an injury, the statute of limitations may be tolled. He may assume there will be no lasting harm to the patient but sometimes that is not the case. The relatively short one or two years for the patient to file a lawsuit may be extended by the non-disclosure.

Whether a disclosure is made as part of a larger hospital team or privately by the doctor, the issue often arises whether the doctor should apologize for the event. Historically such expression of contrition was frowned on by the medical and legal community for fear it would embolden litigation. "Deny and defend" was the mantra. As apology has become more common, in the last few years about half of the states have enacted laws preventing patients from using a doctor's apology as an admission of guilt or legal responsibility. Whether saying "I'm sorry" prevents the filing of lawsuits is still up for debate.

As a general proposition, a carefully worded expression of "regret" or "sorrow for the loss" is not an admission of legal fault or wrong-doing. It should rightfully be viewed as an appropriate expression of compassionate empathy for the suffering of one's patient. If the facts warrant, it can even be accompanied by a statement the situation was "unavoidable" or "unpreventable." All doctors are encouraged to consult local legal counsel how best to proceed with an apology. As author Mark Twain advised: "Do the right thing. It will gratify some people and astonish the rest!"

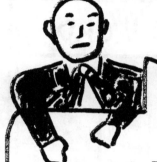

Do This

Become familiar with the 29 "never" events

Follow your institution's disclosure policy

Inform patients of all impactful health events

Keep all disclosures truthful and factual

Express sympathy or sorrow as appropriate

Don't Do This

Avoid talking to the patient/family

Blame others or speculate about causes

Think written disclosure alone is sufficient

Extend litigation times by hiding information

Fail to document a disclosure

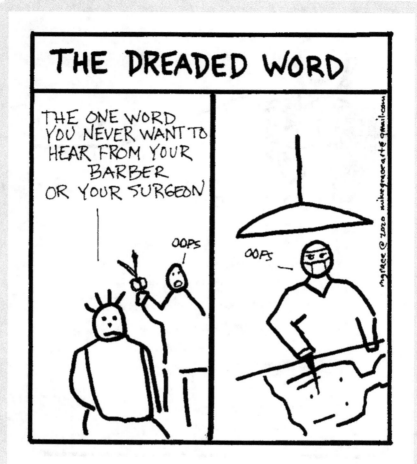

35
Terminating the Relationship

IN THIS CHAPTER

Patients and doctors learn they have a right to terminate the doctor-patient relationship at any time. However, doctors are reminded there are professional and ethical requirements for the timing and manner of the termination.

Both the doctor and the patient can terminate the relationship. As we've seen in the Patient Bill of Rights, the patient has the right to choose a health-care provider. Implied is the right to fire one at any time.

It is considerably trickier for the doctor. There are ethical obligations for how the message is communicated and when.[62] Here are the salient points to keep in mind:

- The doctor may never abandon the patient. Emergency services must be rendered. Non-emergencies should be postponed.
- The doctor may terminate the relationship for any reason—non-payment of a bill, lack of compliance with the agreed treatment plan, or a breakdown in interpersonal communication, to name a few.
- Keep in mind the patient who has discharged himself from the hospital against medical advice (AMA) has not terminated the doctor-patient relationship in most jurisdictions unless the doctor is an employee of the hospital.

---

[62] American Medical Association, "Terminating a Patient-Physician Relationship," Opinion E-1.1.5

- Notification of the termination of the relationship should be communicated verbally but always must be confirmed in writing. Best practice is to send the notification "return receipt requested" so there is future proof the message was sent and received.
- Don't identify a reason. It is sufficient to say words to the effect: "This letter is intended to notify you I am terminating our doctor-patient relationship. I will no longer be available to render medical care and treatment to you effective (date)". Unless you're retiring, offering reasons only invites rebuttal. You have already decided to end the relationship and no purpose is served by hearing the patient argue he indeed followed your medical advice.
- The letter should identify a specific date when the relationship will end. You can never say "effective immediately," no matter how quickly you want to wash your hands of the patient! Best practice is at least three weeks. The idea is to give the patient a reasonable amount of time to find a new provider.
- You must be available to take care of the patient during the three-week interval. You should assure the patient in writing there will be on-going care while he secures a new doctor.
- There must be a continuity of care. Offer to have a copy of the patient's medical chart forwarded to the new provider as soon as she has been identified and offer to speak with her if desired. Of course, should there be a conversation, avoid saying anything negative about the patient. Best to attribute the decision simply to a "breakdown in the relationship."
- Contrary to the old song, breaking up should NOT be hard to do. Not every relationship is a good fit. Either party should feel free to move on!.

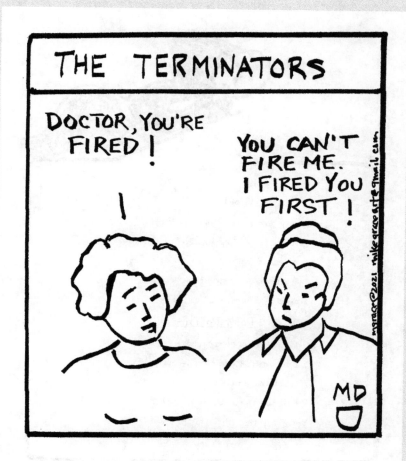

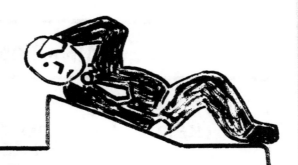

Do This

Change doctors, hospitals or patients if you like

Give the patient fair time to find another doctor

Send written notice "return receipt requested"

Provide emergency services as needed

Provide care during the "waiting period"

Don't Do This

Think patient or doctor needs a reason

End the relationship "effective immediately"

Abandon the patient without care continuity

Refuse to copy records for the patient

Bad mouth the patient to the new doctor.

References and Resources

Chapter 1—Where We Are

The Joint Commission, "JC sentinel event data, root causes by event type 2004–2013," 2014 Oct 1, https://www.jointcommission.org/assets

Cooke, M., "TeamSTEPPS for health care risk managers: Improving teamwork and communication," ASHRM Journal of Healthcare Risk Management, 2016; 36(3): 35, 36

Gilligan, C., Brubacher, S., Powell, M., "Assessing the training needs of medical students in patient information gathering," BMC Medical Education, 2020; 20: 61

CRICO Strategies, "Malpractice risk in communication failures," 2015 Annual Benchmarking Report, Boston, MA: The Risk Management Foundation of the Harvard Medical Institutions, Inc., 2015

Beckman, H.B., Markakis, K.M., Suchman, A.L., Frankel, R.M., "The doctor-patient relationship and malpractice. Lessons from plaintiff depositions," Arch Intern Med, 1994; 154: 1365–1370

Back, A., Fromme, E., Meier, D., "Training Clinicians with Communication Skills Needed to Match Medical Treatments to Patient Values," Journal of the American Geriatrics Society, 2019 May; 67(52): 1, 3

Wilson, B., et al., "Is experience a good teacher? How interns and attending physicians understand patients' choices for end-of-life care," Medical Decision Making, 1997 April–Jun; 17(2): 217–27

Chapter 2—We Once Knew It All

Morin, A., "Important Social Skills for First Grade," Very Well Family, 2020 Sept 17, https://www.verywellfamily.com/social-skills-that-are-important-for-1st-grade-620955

Haq, C., Steele, D., Marchand, L., Seibert, C., Brody, D., "Integrating the Art and Science of Medical Practice: Innovations in Teaching Medical Communications Skills," Family Medicine, 2004 Jan; 36 Suppl: S43

Texas Essential Knowledge and Skills for Grade1, "Section 110.3 English Language Arts and Reading, Grade 1, Adopted 2017," https://www.tea.texas.gov

First Grade Standards for the State of California, "Grade One Standards in Language Arts: Listening and Speaking 1.0 Listening and Speaking Strategies," https://www.teachingfirst.net/standardsfirst.htm

Chapter 3—The Importance of a Name

Davis, L., "The Power of Using Someone's Name," The Native Idealist, 2017 Aug 10, https://www.goodmenproject.com/featured-content/the-power-of-using-someones-name-Idvs/

Russell, J., "Career Coach: The power of using a name," The Washington Post, 2014 Jan 12

Chapter 4—Handshakes and Other Greetings

Center for Disease Control (CDC), "Keeping the workplace safe," 2019, https://www.cdc.gov/coronavirus/2019-ncov/downloads/workplace-school-and-home

Kozlowski, L., Kiviniemi, M., and Ram, P., "Easier Said Than Done: Behavioral Conflicts in Following Social-Distancing Recommendations for Influenza Prevention," Public Health Reports, 2010 Nov–Dec; 125(6): 789–792

Younis, O., "Hello, social distancing. Goodbye, handshakes?", Reuters, 2020 April 28, https://www.reuters.com/article/us-health-coronavirus-handshakes-hello-social-distancing-goodbye-handshakes-idUSKCN22A1D3

Chapter 5—A Communication Model

Joint Commission Resources, "All 8 Models of Communication, Explained!" 2020, https://www.helpfulprofessor.com/communication-models/

Gavi, Z., "The Models of Communication," The Communication Process, 2013 Aug 19, https://www.thecommunicationprocess.com/models-of-communication/

Chapter 6—Interruption

Phillips, K., Ospina, N., Montori, V., "Physicians Interrupting Patients," Journal of General Internal Medicine, 2019 Oct; 34(10): 1965

Rhoades, D., McFarland, K., Finch, W., Johnson, A., "Speaking and interruptions during primary care office visits," Family Medicine, 2001 July–Aug; 33(7): 528–32

Phillips, K., Ospina, N., "Physicians Interrupting Patients," JAMA, 2007; 318(1): 93–94

Chapter 7—Technical Talk

Killian, L., Coletti, M., "The role of universal health literacy precautions in minimizing 'medspeak' and promoting shared decision making," AMA J Ethics, 2017; 19(3): 296–303

O'Reilly, K., "The ABCs of health literacy," American Medical News, 2012 March 19, American Medical Association, https://www.amednews.com

Agency for Healthcare Research and Quality (AHRQ), Health Literacy Toolkit, 2017

Chapter 8—Patient Barriers to Understanding

Safeer, R., Keenan, J., "Health Literacy: The Gap Between Physicians and Patients," Am Fam Physician, 2005 Aug 1; 72(3): 463–468

The Joint Commission, "Ambulatory Health Care National Patient Safety Goals, NPSG.03.06.01," 2020

Agency for Healthcare Research and Quality (AHRQ), "Health Literacy: Hidden Barriers and Practical Strategies," 2015

Beagley, L., "Educating Patients: Understanding Barriers, Learning Styles, and Teaching Techniques," Journal of PeriAnesthesia Nursing, 2011 Oct; 26(5): 331–337

Cochrane, L., Olson, C., et al., "Gaps between knowing and doing: Understanding and assessing the barriers to optimal health care," Journal of Continuing Education in the Health Professions, 2007 June 18; 27(2): 1–8

Chapter 9—It's More About Listening

Tayal, S., Michelson, K., Tayal, N., "Empathetic Listening," AMA STEPS Forward, 2016 Aug 31, https://www.edhub.ama-assn.org/steps-forward/module/2702561

O'Connor, M., "Empathizing with narrative medicine," Hospitals & Health Networks (H&HN), 2017 Oct; 10

Chapter 10—Human Barriers to Active Listening

Mager, D., "The 4 Primary Principles of Communication," Psychology Today, 2007 Feb 13, https://www.psychologytoday.com/us/blog/some-assembly-required201702/the-4-primary-principles-communication

Swayden, K., Anderson, K., et al., "Effect of sitting vs. standing on perception of provider time at bedside: a pilot study," Patient Educ Couns, 2012 Feb; 86(2): 166–171

Navarro, J., Karlins, M., *What Every Body Is Saying*, (Collins) 2008

Yaffe, P., "The 7% Rule—Fact, Fiction, or Misunderstanding," Ubiquity, 2011 Oct; 1–5

Marcinowicz, L., Konstantynowicz, J., Godlewski, C., "Patients' perceptions of GP non-verbal communication: a qualitative study," British Journal of General Practice, 2010; 60(571): 83–87

Nguyen, T., "You Don't Say? Body Language Speaks Volumes More Than Words," Entrepreneur, 2014 November 24, https://www.entrepreneur.com/article/239831

Chapter 11—Physical Barriers to Active Listening

Gaffey, A., Groves, S., "The Clinical Record," In Carroll, R. (ed), *Risk Management Handbook for Healthcare Organizations*, 6th edition, 2011; 331, 355

Zainab, K., "Effects of exam room EHR use on doctor-patient communication: a systematic literature review," Inform Prim Care, 2013; 21(1): 30–39

McGrath, J., Nedal, H., Arar, J., Pugh J., "The Influence of electronic medical record usage on nonverbal communication in the medical interview," Health Informatics Journal, 2017 June 1, https://www.doi.org/10.1177/1460458207076466

Frankel, R., Altschuler, A., George, S., et al., "Effects of exam-room computing on clinician-patient communication," J Gen Intern Med, 2005; 20: 677–682, https://www.doi.org/10.1111/j.1525-1497.2005.0163.x

Russell, S., "An Overview of Adult-Learning," Urologic Nursing, 2006 Oct; 26(5): 349, 370

BaRoss, C., "Designing for Health: Responding to Shifting Patient Demographics Through Empathic Design," Contrack Design Network, 2015 Sept 14, https://www.contractdesign.com/practice/healthcare/designing-for-health-responding-to-shifting-patient-demographics-through-empathic-design/

Chapter 12—Nurse-Doctor Communication

Jessie, C., "How To Build a Better Doctor Nurse Relationship," Med Study, 2020 May 6, https://www.mkt.medstudy.com/glog/how-to-build-better-doctor-nurse-relationship

Siediecki, S., Hixson, E., "Relationships Between Nurses and Physicians Matter," The Online Journal of Issues in Nursing, 2015 Aug 31; 20(3)

Benner, A., "Physician and nurse relationships, a key to patient safety," J Ky Med Assoc, 2007; 105(4): 165–169

Gallup Politics, "Nurses Again Outpace Other Professions for Honesty, Ethics," Dec 20, 2018, https://www.news.gallup.com/pdf/245597/nurses-again-outpace

Roberts, S., DeMarco, R., and Griffin, M., "The Effect of Oppressed Group Behaviors on the Culture of the Nursing Workplace: A Review of the Evidence and Interventions for Change," *Journal of Nursing Management*, 2009; 17: 288–293

Hutchinson, M., Vickers, M., Jackson, D., Wilkes, L., "Workplace Bullying in Nursing: Toward a Moe Critical Organizational Perspective," *Nursing Inquiry*, 2006; 13(2): 118–126

Bartholomew, K., "Ten Steps to Improving Physician-Nurse Relationships," https://www.marylandpatientsafety.org/html/education/0402091/document/130-Rm321-23a.pdf.

Bartholomew, K., *Speak Your Truth: Proven Strategies for Effective Nurse-Physician Communication*, 2005

Shaneela, S., Sumesh, T., "Situation, Background, Assessment, Recommendation (SBAR) Communication Tool for Handoff in Health Care-A Narrative Review," Safety in Health, 2018; 4(7): 2–5

Larson, J., "Five Ways to Promote Healthy Nurse-Doctor Relationships," Nursing, 2017; 37(1): 52–55

Institute for Healthcare Improvement, "SBAR: Situation-Background-Assessment-Recommendation," 2017 (The SBAR tool was developed by Kaiser Permanente). https://www.ihi.org

Chapter 13—Communication Within Teams

Roberts, K., Yu, K., van Stralen, D., "Patient safety is an organizational systems issue: lessons from a variety of industries." In Youngberg, B. and Hatlie, M. (eds.) *The Patient Safety Handbook*, Canada: Jones and Bartlett, 2004

Reason, J., *Human Error,* Cambridge: Cambridge University Press, 1990

Schwartz, M., et al., "The effects of crew resource management on teamwork and safety climate at Veterans Health Administration facilities," ASHRM Journal of Healthcare Risk Management, 2018; 38(1); 17–37

De Leval, M., "Human factors and surgical outcomes: A Cartesian dream," Lancet, 1997; 349(9053): 723–725

Chapter 14—The Testimonial

Levinson, W., "Doctor-patient communication and medical malpractice: implications for pediatricians," Pediatric Annals, 1997 Feb 28; 26(3): 186–193

Stone, J., "The Importance of Empathy in Healthcare: Advancing Humanism," Medical GPS, 2019

CRICO Strategies, "Malpractice risk in communication failures," 2015 Annual Benchmarking Report, Boston, MA: The Risk Management Foundation of the Harvard Medical Institutions, Inc., 2015

Huntington, B., "Communication Gaffes: a root cause of malpractice claims," Proceedings, (Baylor Univ Medical Center), 2003 April; 16(2): 157–161

Shapiro, R., "A Survey of sued and non-sued physicians and suing patients," Arch Internal Medicine, 1989; 149(2): 190–196

Siegel, D., "Harnessing the power of medical malpractice data to improve patient care," ASHRM Journal of Healthcare Risk Management, 2019 Nov; 39(3): 31

Association of American Medical Colleges, Report 1-Learning Objectives for Medical Student Education-Guidelines for Medical Schools, 1998 Jan; 4–6

Chapter 15—Patient Preparation for the Office Visit

US Dept of Health & Human Services, National Institute on Aging, "How to Prepare for a Doctor's Appointment," www.nia.nih.gov/health/how-prepare-doctors-appointment

Cleveland Clinic, "5 Ways to Make the Most of Your Doctor's Appointment," 2020 Sept 16, www.health.clevelandclinic.org/5-ways-to-make-the-most-of-your-doctors-appointment/

Chapter 16—Patient Preparation for the Hospital Stay

The Joint Commission, "Inadequate hand-off communication," Sentinel Alert Event, Issue 58, 2017 Sept 12

Agency for Healthcare Research and Quality (AHRQ), "Strategy 6G: Training to Advance Physicians' Communication Skills," 2017 July, https://www.ahrq.gov/sites/default/files/wysiwyg/cahps/quality-improvement/improvement-guide/6-strategies-for-improvement

Robeznieks, A., "Successful Handoff? A good discharge planning process follows a patient across the continuum of care from hospital to home," Hospitals and Health Networks (H&HN), 2017 June; 41–43

American Medical Association, "Patient Responsibilities," Opinion E-1.1.4

Chapter 17—The Angry Patient

Huntington, B., "Communication Gaffes: a root cause of malpractice claims," Proceedings, (Baylor Univ Medical Center), 2003 April; 16(2): 157, 159

Wible, P., "Waiting Room Remedy: Doctor Pays for Delays (The Doctor's Perspective)," J. Participat Med, 2012 Jan; 11(4): e1

National Academy of Sciences, *Issues in Access, Scheduling, and Wait Times—Transforming Health Care Scheduling and Access*, 2015, https://www.ncbi.nlm.nih.gov/books/NBK3316141/

Petrow, S., "My doctor kept me waiting forever. Can I get some sort of refund?", The Washington Post, 2018 Jan 20

Chapter 18—The Quiet Patient

Tayal, S., Michelson, K., Tayal, N., "Empathetic Listening," AMA STEPS Forward, 2016 Aug 31, https://www.dhub.ama-assn.org/steps-forward/module/2702561

National Center for Health Statistics, *Summary Health Statistics Tables for U.S. Adults: National Health Interview Survey, 2018*, Table A-18c

National Center for Health Statistics, *Summary Health Statistics Tables for U.S. Children: national Health Interview Survey, 2018*, Table C-8c

National Center for Health Statistics, *Utilization of Ambulatory Medical Care by Women: United States, 1997–1998*, Series Report 13, No. 149

Watt, D., "The Guys' Guide to Doctor Visits," One Medical, 2019 Nov 19, https://www.onemedical.com/blog/live-well/guys-doctor-guide

Chapter 19—The Unfocused Patient

Schulz, J., "Using a person's name in conversation," Michigan State University Extension, 2017 Jan 12

Tesema, M., "4 Science-Backed Reasons to Say Your Self—Talk Out Loud," Shine, 2020 Sept 18, https://www.advice.theshineapp.com/articles/4/science-backed-reasons-to-take-your-self-talk-out-loud/

Chapter 20—The Patient's Family

Hickson, O., Chayton, E., Githens, P., Sloan, F., "Factors that prompted families to file medical malpractice claims following perinatal injuries," JAMA, 1992; 267: 1359–1363

Vincent, C., Young, M., Phillips, A., "Why do people sue doctors? A study of patients and relatives taking legal action," Lancet, 1994; 343: 1609–1663

McClellan, F., "Do Poor People Sue Doctors More Frequently? Confronting Unconscious Bias and the Role of Cultural Competency," *Clinical Orthopaedics and Related Research*, 2012 May

"How doctors can spot patients likely to sue," American Medical News, amedmews. com, 2013 Feb 4

Siegel, D., "Harnessing the power of medical malpractice data to improve patient care," ASHRM Journal of Healthcare Risk Management, 2019 Nov; 39(3): 36

Chapter 21—Legal Healthcare Documents

American Bar Association, "Giving Someone a Power of Attorney for Your Healthcare (multi-state guide and form)," 2020 Aug 25, https://www.americanbar. org/groups/law_aging/resources/health_care_decsion_making/power__atty_ guide_and_form_2011

McCarrick, P., "Living Will and Durable Power of Attorney Advance Directive Legislation and Issues," National Reference Center for Bioethics Literature Georgetown University, 2001, https://www.bioethics.georgetown.edu

Chapter 22—The Patient Bill of Rights

CMS Manual System Department of Health & Human Services (DHHS), Centers for Medicare & Medicaid. Services (CMS), Pub. 100-07 State Operations, Provider Certification Transmittal 37, 2008 October 17

Privacy Act of 1974 (2020 edition), 5 USC, Section 552A, Individual's Right of Amendment (2–4) found online at www.justice.gov/opcl/privstat.htm

Hanauer, D., Preib, R., Zheng, K., Choi, S., "Patient-initiated electronic health record amendment requests," J Am Med Inform Assoc, 2014 Nov–Dec; (6): 992–1000, https://pubmed.ncbi.nlm.nih.gov/24863430/

Centers for Medicare and Medicaid, Conditions of Participation, Patient Rights, 42 CFR 482.13(b)(2)

American Medical Association, "Patient Rights," Opinion E-1.1.3

Chapter 23—The Disabled Patient

California Medical Association, "ADA/Discrimination," *California Physician's Legal Handbook*, 2004; 1: 1–79

Title III of the Americans with Disabilities ACT (1990), Section 504 of the Rehabilitation Act (1973)

National League for Nursing, "Communicating with People with Disabilities," https://www.nln.org/professional-development-programs/teaching-resources/ace-d/additional-resources/communicating-with-people-with-disabilities#

Center for Disease Control and Prevention (CDC), "Communicating With and About People with Disabilities," 2020 Sept 16

North Dakota Center for Persons with Disability, "Communicating Effectively With People Who Have A Disability," https://www.ndcpd.org

Chapter 24—The Foreign Patient

The Joint Commission (TJC), *A Crosswalk of the National Standards for Culturally and Linguistically Appropriate Services (CLAS) in Health and Health Care*, 2014

Title VI Civil Rights Act of 1964, Executive Order 13166, Section 1557 of the Patient Protection and Affordable Care ACT

Carrillo, J., "Cross-cultural primary care: A patient-based approach," Ann Intern Med, 1999, May 18; 130(10): 829–34

Crisp, A., Edwards, W., "Communication in medical practice across ethnic boundaries," Postgraduate Medical Journal, 1989; 65: 150–155

Singleton, K., Krause, E., "Understanding Cultural and Linguistic Barriers to Health Literacy," The Online Journal of Issues in Nursing (OJIN), 2009 Sept 30; 14(3)

Chapter 25—Informed Consent

American Society for Healthcare Risk Management (ASHRM), *Informed Consent and the Law*, Chicago: American Society for Healthcare Risk Management, 2000

Centers for Medicare and Medicaid, Conditions of Participation, Surgical Services, 42 CFR 482.51 (b)(2)

CMS Memorandum, April 13, 2007, "Revisions to the Hospital Interpretive Guidelines for Informed Consent."

Cobbs v Grant (1972) 8 Cal 3rd 229 (This is the California Supreme Court landmark decision on informed consent.)

Truman v. Thomas (1980) 27 Cal 3rd 285 (This is the follow-up California Supreme Court decision extending the physician's duty of informed consent to medical treatment and diagnostic tests.)

Chapter 26—Conduct During Examinations

North Carolina Medical Board, Guidelines for Avoiding Misunderstandings During Patient Encounters and Physical Examinations, 1991, Amended Mar 2019, https://www.ncmedboard.org/resources-information/professional-resources/laws-rules-position-statements/position-statements/guidelines_for_avoiding

Hooper, C., "What is a Physical Exam and What Can You Expect?" Dignity Health, 2017 May 2, https://www.dignityhealth.org/articles/what-is-a-physical-exam-and-what-can-you-expect

Chapter 27—Communicating in the Medical Record

Gaffey, A., Groves, S., "The Clinical Record," In Carroll, R. (ed) *Risk Management Handbook for Healthcare Organizations*, 6th edition, 2011; 331–365

Day, N. *The Medical Record, Your Best Friend or Worst Enemy*. American College of Healthcare Administration, 1998; 9–13

Seegert, L., "5 Strategies to reduce malpractice lawsuit threats," 2016 Nov 10, https://www.medicaleconomics.com

Dougherty, M., "Maintaining a Legally Sound Health Record," Journal of AHIMA, 2003 April; 73(8): 64A-G, https://www.ahima.org

Chapter 28—Confidentiality

The Health Insurance Portability and Accountability Act (HIPAA) of 1996, https://www.hhs.gov/ocr/hipaa

American Medical Association, "Confidentiality-Code of Medical Ethics Opinion 3.2.1," https://www.ama-assn.org/delivering-care/ethics/confidentiality

Tariz, R., Hackert, P., Patient Confidentiality. 2020 Aug 22. In: StatPearls [Internet]. Treasure Island (FL): StatPearls Publishing; 2020 Jan-. PMID: 30137825

Chapter 29—Sex Talk

Rizza, S., MacGowan, R., et al., "HIV Screening in the Health Care Setting: Status, Barriers, and Potential Solutions," Symposium on Antimicrobial Therapy, 2012 Sept 1; 87(9): 1–34

National District Attorneys' Association, *Minor Consent to Medical Treatment Laws*, 2013

Jayasuriya, A., Dennick, R., "Sexual history-taking; using educational interventions to overcome barriers to learning," Sex Education, 2011; 11(1): 99–112

Wiskin, C., Roberts, L., Roalfe, A., "The impact of discussing a sexual history in role-play simulation teaching on pre-clinical student attitudes towards people who submit for STI testing," Medical Teacher, 2011; 33(6): 324–32

Chapter 30—The Transgender and Non-Binary Patient

The University of Iowa Healthcare, "Quick tips for medical providers of transgender patients-The Transcare approach," https://www.uihc.org/health-topics/quick-tips-medical-providers-transgender-patients

Steuer, K., Davis, K., "Respecting Gender Identity in Healthcare: Regulatory Requirements and Recommendations for Treating Transgender Patients," The Health Lawyer, 2017 Feb; 29(3): 1, 3–9, https://www.amicanbar.org/groups/gpsolo/publications/gpsolo_ereport/2017/respecting_gender_identity_healthcare_regulatory_requirements

Kelly, M., *Providing Transgender and Non-Binary Care at Planned Parenthood*, 2018; 41–43 (citing documents from The American Academy of Pediatrics, American Academy of Physician Assistants, The American College of Obstetricians and Gynecologists (ACOG), The American Medical Association, The American Psychological Association, The American Public Health Association, and The Endocrine Society) and at 27–28 (citing the 2015 U.S. Transgender Survey (USTS))

Center for Disease Control and Prevention (CDC), "Patient-Centered Care for Transgender People: Recommended Practices for Health Care Settings," 2020 April 1

Goldhammer, H., Malina, S., Seurogblian, A., "Communicating With Patients Who Have Nonbinary Gender Identities," Annals of Fam Med, 2018 Nov/Dec; 16(6): 559–562

Chapter 31—The Elderly Patient

Robinson, T., "Improving Communication With Older Patients: Tips From the Literature," Fam Pract Manag, 2006 Sept; 13(8): 73–78

Weiss, C., "Fall Prevention Among the Elderly," 2002 June, https://www.nursingspectrum.com

US Dept of Health & Human Services, National Institute on Aging, "Tips for Improving Communication with Older Patients," 2017 May 17, https://www.nia.nih.gov/health/tips-improving-communication-older-patients

O'Connor, M., "The future of age-friendly care," Hospitals & Health Network (H&HN), 2017 March; 13

Chapter 32—The Seriously Ill Patient

Gregory, C., "The Five Stages of Grief-An Examination of the Kubler-Ross Model," Psycom, https://www.psycom.net/authors/christina-gregory-phd

Riecke, P., *How to Talk with Sick, Dying, and Grieving People*, 2018: 77

Headly, A., "Communication Skills: A Call for Teaching to the Test," American Journal of Medicine, 2007 Oct 1; 120(10): 910–915; https://www.amjmed.com/article/S0002-9343(07)00726-7/fulltext

Back, A., Fromme, E., Meier, D., "Training Clinicians with Communication Skills Needed to Match Medical Treatments to Patient Values," Journal of the American Geriatrics Society, 2019 May; 67(52): 1, 9

Curtis, J., Patrick, D., Caldwell, E., Collier, A., "Why Don't Patients and Physicians Talk About End-of Life Care? Barriers to Communication for Patients With Acquired Immunodeficiency Syndrome and Their Primary Care Clinicians," Arch Intern Med, 2000; 160(11): 1690–1696

Chapter 33—Telemedicine

U.S. Department of Health & Human Services, "Notification of Enforcement Discretion for Telehealth Remote Communications During the COVID-19 Nationwide Public Health Emergency," https://www.hhs.gov/hipaa/for-professionals/special-topics/emergency-preparedness/notification-enforcement-discretion-telehealth/index.html

American Medical Association, "Ethical Practice in Telemedicine," Opinion E-1.2.12

American Association of Healthcare Risk Management (ASHRM), Telemedicine (white paper), 2018; Russell, D., (ed)

Chapter 34—Doctor Disclosure and Apology

National Quality Forum (NQF), *Serious Reportable Event in Healthcare—2011 Update: A Consensus Report*, Washington, DC: NQF; 2011

Leapfrog, "When hospitals and surgery centers say 'I'm sorry,'" https://www.leapfroggroup.org/influencing/never-events

ACOG Committee Opinion 380: "Disclosure and discussion of adverse events." ACOG committee on Quality Improvement and Patient Safety and Committee on Professional Liability. Obstet Gynecol. 2007; 1(10): 957–958

Risk Management Pearls on Disclosure of Adverse Events, Chicago. ASHRM, 2011. Available at https://www.ashrmstore.org

Popp, P., "How will disclosure affect future litigation?" ASHRM Journal of Healthcare Risk Management, 2003; 131(23): 963–967

Mazor, K., Simon, S., Gurwitz, J., "Communicating with patients about medical errors: a review of the literature." Archives of Internal Medicine, 2004 Aug 9; 164(15): 1690–97

Chapter 35—Terminating the Relationship

American Medical Association, "Terminating a Patient-Physician Relationship," Opinion E-1.1.5

California Medical Association, "Termination of the Physician-Patient Relationship," *California Physician's Legal Handbook*, 2004; 32: 23–31

Acknowledgements

I was blessed at an early age to recognize and pursue my life's two great professional passions—communication and healthcare. The strands of my life quickly came together in a recognizable pattern from high school forensic champ, to college communication major, to medical malpractice trial lawyer, to invited healthcare lecturer, to hospital administrative officer, and now university nurse instructor.

As I was interacting with doctors, nurses and patients over the years, I was regularly struck by how many of the problems in healthcare had miscommunication at the source. The idea of this book began to germinate but the sprouts of a book never took root in the hustle of more immediately pressing responsibilities.

And then came Covid. Amidst the tragedy of a global pandemic, a silver lining was found. Suddenly quarantine and social restrictions gave me the time to commit thoughts to paper. *The Mumbo Jumbo Fix* was born! It is my hope the subtitle, *A Survival Guide for Effective Doctor-Patient-Nurse Communication* is predictive of the benefits this handbook will provide. At least I hope the reader agrees with comedian and author Steve Martin: "I think I did pretty well, considering I started out with nothing but a bunch of blank paper."

I've never aspired to write an academic treatise. My temperament is too practical and my patience too limited for such a scholarly endeavor. The goal was something short, to the point, and fun. That was the inspiration for the cartoons. While I do paint and, in fact, consider myself a portrait painter, the reader will rightly assume this was my first foray into cartoon illustration. My life-long respect and admiration for Charles Schulz and Gary Larson have only deepened!

This project would not have been possible without the support of my partner, Chris Dodson, who kept my creative juices flowing. He thankfully gave me the mental and physical space to work, and the thoughtful feedback I needed.

Special thanks are also due my former law partner, Graham Hollis, and his wife Jasmina. Their intelligence, humor, and wise counsel gave me inspiration and encouragement.

Many other people are also deserving of recognition—Jeremy Blanger for the design of the cover; Elsa Murdoch, DNP, MSN, RN and Eric Hunsgate, M.D. for invaluable nursing and doctor perspectives; Catherine Silber for sharing a lifetime of communication; and Don Shultz for his patient editing and suggested corrections.

As the saying goes, the faults are mine alone. But hopefully I have not added more linguistic mumbo jumbo to the mix.

Mike Grace
Palm Springs, California